DECODING VITALITY

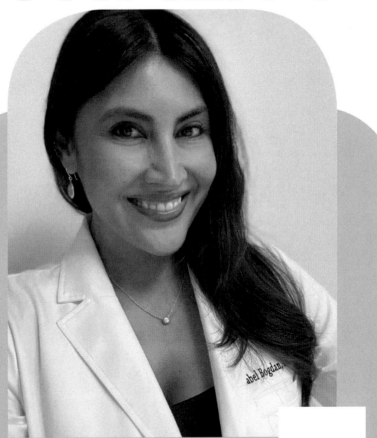

Understand Your Unique Body Code
For A More Vital Body, Mind and Life

belev.co
modern women's health

Dr. Isabel Bogdan

Balboa Press books may be ordered through booksellers or by contacting:

Balboa Press
A Division of Hay House
1663 Liberty Drive
Bloomington, IN 47403
www.balboapress.com
844-682-1282

ISBN: 979-8-7652-5214-7 (sc)
979-8-7652-5280-2 (hc)
979-8-7652-5211-6 (e)

Library of Congress Control Number: 2024910775

Print information available on the last page.

Balboa Press rev. date: 06/19/2024

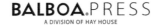

BALBOA.PRESS
A DIVISION OF HAY HOUSE

Contents

Prologue

This book serves as a guiding light for empowering women's health in a world where women's well-being is often overlooked or misunderstood. Isabel Bogdan, DNP, WHNP, a women's health nurse practitioner with a degree specializing in supporting perimenopausal women, brings a wealth of experience, compassion, and expertise to these pages.

As you journey through these chapters, you will embark on a path toward taking charge of your health during the perimenopausal stage.

Isabel's commitment to caring and providing evidence-based practices shines through in her advice, empowering strategies, and deep understanding of women's unique challenges during this pivotal phase of life.

Get ready to be enlightened, motivated, and empowered as you dive into the contents of this book.

Whether you are personally navigating the intricacies of perimenopause or seeking to support someone dear through this experience, the wisdom shared within these pages will illuminate the way toward health and well-being.

This book offers empowerment, knowledge, and encouragement to all women embracing the journey of perimenopause.

Preface

The art of women's health and the hybrid clinician is like a tapestry woven with threads of resilience, complexity, and beauty. Women's health goes beyond well-being, encompassing mental and spiritual harmony. It's more than treatments; it takes a holistic approach that respects each woman's individual path.

Central to women's health is understanding the connection between mind, body, and spirit. True health isn't about being disease-free but about having vitality, balance, and empowerment. From years to menopause, women face changes, obstacles, and victories that shape their health and wellness.

As caretakers of families, community nurturers, and sources of strength, women often prioritize others' needs over their own. The art of women's health encourages them to reclaim control over their lives, focus on self-care, and develop self-awareness. It honors the wisdom and intuition that guide women toward wholeness and vitality.

By exploring the art of women's health, we embark on a journey that values women's needs, experiences, and voices. Through education, empowerment initiatives, and advocacy efforts, we strive to create a world where every woman can flourish and realize her potential.

Come along with me as we explore the complexities of women's health, honor the strength of the essence, and cherish the practice of promoting wellness in every aspect.

The hybrid healthcare provider

A women's health nurse practitioner (WHNP) is an advanced practice registered nurse who delivers holistic healthcare to women of all ages. These trained experts support and enhance women's health and wellness by addressing their distinct healthcare requirements.

Women's health nurse practitioners are skilled in evaluating, diagnosing, and treating women's health issues, such as health, gynecological care, prenatal and postpartum care, menopausal support, and more. They collaborate closely with women to create care plans that cater to their emotional and social well-being. Aside from conducting examinations and screenings, WHNPs offer health education, guidance, and encouragement to empower women to make informed choices about their well-being. They have the authority to prescribe medications, request tests, and perform procedures within their professional scope of practice.

An essential aspect of the work of women's health nurse practitioners (WHNPs) is their focus on care and promoting health and wellness.

By encouraging conversations, establishing trust, and providing an environment for women to talk about their health issues, Women's Health Nurse Practitioners (WHNPs) play a crucial role in empowering women to take charge of their health and overall wellness.

Overall, women's health nurse practitioners serve as advocates, educators, and partners in care for women of all ages. Their dedication to promoting women's health, providing compassionate care, and addressing the unique needs of each individual makes them invaluable members of the healthcare team. The needs of each individual make them invaluable members of the healthcare team.

Chapter One:

Grasping the Concept of how Perimenopause Influences Genetic Makeup, Hormones, and Body Processes

What is Perimenopause?

"I could see the panic set in as beads of sweat began to accumulate on her face, her skin began to flush as she ran to her bedroom and slammed the door shut. I could hear her crying, my mother had a terrible time during her perimenopausal years. I was only seven years old when she was 42, I felt it was my responsibility to help her heal from "whatever" was happening to her - the hot flashes, the mood swings, the joint pain, the booze…the list goes on. I remember the both of us visiting different types of doctors, internal medicine, rheumatology, psychiatrists, and no one was able to help her feel better. Running out of options and trying to connect the pieces, she finally visited with a true healer, someone who sat down to listen to her story. Her blood was drawn and the following day my mother was appropriately diagnosed with a thyroid condition exacerbated by perimenopause and the hormonal changes that happen in midlife. She was given a prescription for thyroid hormone, exercise, and nutrition, me as a bystander and advocate of my mother's care, at such a young age helped her stay accountable, and this is my calling and ministry to you."

- Isabel Bogdan.

Perimenopause marks a phase in a woman's life typically occurring from her 30s to early 50s leading up to menopause. This period involves shifts as estrogen levels fluctuate and eventually decrease, bringing about symptoms like irregular periods, hot flashes, mood swings, and weight changes. It's essential to grasp the effects of perimenopause on your body to navigate this stage effectively.

An essential aspect of perimenopause is its impact on metabolism. With declining estrogen levels, the body's ability to regulate insulin and glucose is affected, resulting in shifts in weight and energy levels. Many women may find it easier to gain weight or challenging to shed pounds during perimenopause due to reduced calorie-burning efficiency. Understanding these metabolic adjustments can help women support their health proactively.

Moreover, perimenopause is linked with heightened inflammation in the body. This inflammation, often called "inflammaging," can worsen discomfort, headaches, and fatigue. Embracing an inflammatory diet emphasizing whole foods rich in nutrients plays a crucial role in managing perimenopausal symptoms.

To help ease the symptoms of perimenopause, women can improve their health by cutting down on processed foods, sugar, and unhealthy fats. It's crucial for women going through perimenopause to prioritize self-care and look after their well-being. Self-care practices like yoga, meditation, or regular exercise can help reduce stress levels. Sleeping and staying hydrated are essential for maintaining balance and metabolism during perimenopause. By taking an approach to their health, women can effectively manage perimenopause symptoms and enhance their overall well-being.

In summary, perimenopause represents a stage in a woman's life marked by fluctuations and metabolic changes. By grasping the essence of perimenopause and its impact on the body, women can take measures to nurture their health and well-being during this period. Embracing an anti-inflammatory diet, prioritizing self-care, and staying physically active is critical in managing perimenopause symptoms and enhancing overall wellness. Equipped with the resources and encouragement, women can confidently navigate perimenopause while setting the stage for a fulfilling future.

Effects of Perimenopause on Metabolism

When women enter perimenopause, their bodies undergo changes that affect their metabolism. These changes can impact health and well-being. Knowing how perimenopause affects metabolism is essential for women looking to stay healthy during this transition period.

A significant way that perimenopause influences metabolism is by decreasing estrogen levels. Estrogen helps regulate metabolism, so as estrogen levels drop during perimenopause, women may notice a change in their metabolic rate. This shift in metabolism can make it harder to manage weight and may lead to weight gain around the waist.

In addition to estrogen level fluctuations, perimenopause can also affect insulin sensitivity. Insulin plays a role in managing blood sugar levels, and changes in insulin sensitivity can impact metabolism. Women experiencing perimenopause might see an increase in insulin resistance, which could result in weight gain and stubborn abdominal fat.

Perimenopause could also cause shifts in muscle mass since women naturally lose muscle as they age, slowing down their metabolism. This loss of muscle mass can occur rapidly during perimenopause, underscoring the importance of incorporating strength training exercises into their workout routine to preserve muscle mass and support metabolism.

It's crucial for women going through perimenopause to grasp how it influences their metabolism.

During perimenopause, women can take control of their metabolism and overall well-being by making choices about their diet, exercise, and lifestyle habits. By adopting approaches and strategies, women can confidently navigate this stage with vitality.

Women must recognize the signs of metabolic changes that occur during perimenopause, as these changes impact health and quality of life at this time. In the following discussion, we will explore some indicators of metabolic shifts in perimenopause and provide insights on managing them through a diet tailored to women's health and a program to reset metabolism.

One common indication of metabolic changes during perimenopause is weight gain around the midsection. This increase in body weight is often associated with fluctuations in insulin, estrogen, and progesterone levels, which can affect metabolism and lead to buildup. One of the biggest confounding variables is a loss of muscle mass and increase of total body fat. By following a diet designed for women's health and participating in a metabolism reset program, individuals can explore ways to improve their choices and lifestyle habits to maintain weight during this transitional phase.

Another prevalent sign of metabolic changes during perimenopause is fatigue, characterized by decreased energy levels. Hormonal imbalances can impact energy production and metabolism, leading to feelings of tiredness and lethargy. Through targeted adjustments, like incorporating foods into their diet and engaging in physical activity, individuals can boost their energy levels and combat the fatigue commonly experienced during perimenopause.

During perimenopause, besides experiencing weight gain and fatigue, many individuals may also notice shifts in their mood and mental well-being. Hormonal changes can lead to mood swings, irritability, and symptoms of anxiety or depression.

To support their well-being during this phase, women can focus on a diet that reduces inflammation, including mood-boosting nutrients, and engage in activities that help reset metabolism while emphasizing stress management techniques.

Common signs of metabolic changes during perimenopause include bloating, gas, constipation, and sleep disruption. These symptoms may be linked to metabolic imbalances. By addressing these issues through lifestyle adjustments and stress management strategies, women can improve their health and sleep quality during perimenopause.

Addressing the signs of metabolic shifts during perimenopause empowers women to take steps to maintain their health throughout this period. Following the Belev approach, which emphasizes nutrition choices, lifestyle habits, and overall well-being, women can navigate perimenopause smoothly and with vitality.

Exploring the Connection between DNA and Metabolism.

What is DNA?

This section will explore DNA and its significance for our health. DNA—acid—is the material carrying instructions for all living organisms' development, functioning, growth, and reproduction.

Think of DNA as instructions containing the information needed to construct and maintain our bodies. Each person's DNA is unique, and it comes from their parents. DNA consists of four chemical elements: adenine, thymine, guanine, and cytosine. They join together like steps on a staircase called a helix. These elements combine (adenine with thymine and guanine with cytosine) to form the blueprint that defines characteristics like eye color, hair type, and predisposition to certain illnesses.

Understanding our DNA is crucial for optimizing our health, especially during perimenopause. Research has shown that certain genetic variations can influence our risk of developing conditions like heart disease, diabetes, and cancer. By knowing our genetic makeup, we can make informed decisions about our lifestyle, diet, and healthcare choices to mitigate these risks and support our overall well-being.

In recent years, technological advances have made accessing information about our DNA through services like genetic testing kits easier and more affordable. These tests can provide valuable insights into our genetic predispositions and help us tailor our health and wellness strategies accordingly. By understanding our genetic profile, we can personalize our approach to diet, exercise, and supplementation to optimize our metabolic health and support our journey through perimenopause.

The Belev method will help you explore how DNA influences our metabolism and how we can use this knowledge to achieve our health goals. By learning about the role of DNA in our bodies and how it can impact our health during perimenopause, we can empower ourselves to make informed choices that support our well-being and vitality. DNA is not just a scientific concept - it is a powerful tool that can help us take control of our health and thrive during this transformative stage of life.

- What you need to know about how your DNA works

With the Belev method, Isabel will help you explore the fascinating world of your DNA and how it plays a crucial role in your health and well-being, especially during the perimenopausal years—understanding how your DNA works can provide valuable insights into how your body responds to different foods, stressors, and lifestyle choices. By unlocking the secrets of your genetic code, you can make more informed decisions about your health and take proactive steps to optimize your metabolism and overall well-being.

Your DNA is like a blueprint that contains all the instructions for building and maintaining your body. It comprises a unique sequence of nucleotides that encode the genes responsible for various biological processes. These genes can influence everything from your metabolism and hormone production to your immune system and inflammation levels. By understanding how your DNA works, you can identify potential genetic predispositions that may impact your health during perimenopause.

A critical aspect of DNA work is gene expression, which refers to the process by which the information stored in your genes is used to create proteins that carry out specific bodily functions. Various factors, including diet, lifestyle, and environment, can influence gene expression. By making strategic choices that support healthy gene expression, you can optimize your metabolism and reduce inflammation, which are critical goals in perimenopause.

Another critical concept to understand about how your DNA works are genetic variations or polymorphisms, which are differences in the genetic code that can affect how your body processes nutrients, detoxifies harmful substances and responds to stress. You can better tailor your diet and lifestyle choices to support your unique genetic makeup by identifying genetic variations that may impact your health. This personalized approach can help you achieve better results with your women's anti-inflammatory diet and metabolic reset course.

In conclusion, knowing how your DNA works is essential for optimizing your health during perimenopause. By understanding the role of gene expression and genetic variations in your metabolism and inflammation levels, you can make more informed choices that support your unique genetic makeup. This personalized approach can help you achieve lasting results with your women's anti-inflammatory diet and metabolic reset course, leading to improved health and well-being as you navigate the challenges of perimenopause.

- How inflammation harms DNA

Inflammation is a natural response by the body to protect itself from harm, but when it becomes chronic, it can damage our DNA. Inflammation is especially concerning for women in perimenopause, as hormonal changes during this time can exacerbate inflammation and increase the risk of developing chronic diseases. Understanding how inflammation harms our DNA is crucial for taking control of our health and preventing long-term damage.

One way inflammation harms DNA is through the production of free radicals. These unstable molecules can cause oxidative stress, which damages DNA and impairs its ability to function correctly. Oxidative stress can lead to mutations and other genetic abnormalities that increase the risk of developing diseases such as cancer, heart disease, and autoimmune disorders. By reducing inflammation through diet and lifestyle changes, we can help protect our DNA from these harmful effects.

Inflammation can also directly impact our DNA's structure, leading to gene expression changes. When inflammatory markers are consistently elevated, they can alter how our genes are read and transcribed, affecting the production of proteins essential for maintaining our health. This dysregulation can contribute to the development of metabolic disorders, hormonal imbalances, and other health issues commonly experienced during perimenopause. By managing inflammation, we can help restore balance to our genetic blueprint and support our overall well-being.

Chronic inflammation can also accelerate the aging process by shortening the length of our telomeres, which are protective caps at the ends of our chromosomes. As telomeres shorten, cells become less able to divide and regenerate, leading to premature aging and an increased risk of age-related diseases. By reducing inflammation and supporting our cellular health, we can help preserve the length of our telomeres and promote longevity during perimenopause and beyond.

In conclusion, understanding how inflammation harms our DNA is essential for women in perimenopause who are seeking to reset their health and prevent chronic diseases. Addressing inflammation through an anti-inflammatory diet, stress management techniques and other lifestyle interventions can protect our DNA from damage, support healthy gene expression, and promote longevity. Taking a proactive approach to managing inflammation can help us navigate the challenges of perimenopause with grace and vitality, empowering us to thrive during this transformative stage of life.

Chapter Two:

Understanding How Inflammation and Cardiometabolic Health Influence Perimenopause

"She was only 12 years old and she was already concerned about her weight, she noticed an increase in bloating and feelings of anxiety around the time of her menstrual cycle. Her periods were heavy, and painful, and usually unpredictable. She was told this was "normal". As years passed, she was diagnosed with polycystic ovary syndrome, later diagnosed with gestational diabetes only to have it show up as Type 2 diabetes in her mid forties. Funny thing is, her friends also share the same story, now they are midlife, and they all agree to feeling unsteady, uncalibrated somehow inside their body, inside their thoughts and perhaps even to the world."

Inflammation is a natural defense mechanism our bodies use to protect against harm and facilitate recovery. However, when inflammation persists over time, it can affect women's well-being during perimenopause. Prolonged inflammation has been associated with health issues like heart disease, diabetes, and autoimmune conditions. Recognizing how inflammation influences our bodies is crucial for maintaining health during the perimenopausal phase.

One significant factor contributing to inflammation in women is hormonal shifts. The decrease in estrogen levels during this period can escalate inflammation throughout the body, leading to symptoms like discomfort, fatigue, and weight changes. Women can effectively manage these symptoms. Enhance their well-being by understanding how hormonal fluctuations can influence inflammation. The food we consume plays a role in regulating the body's response. Certain types of food, such as processed sugars, refined grains, and trans fats, can trigger inflammation, while others, like fruits, vegetables, and healthy fats, can help alleviate it. By adhering to an anti-inflammatory diet plan, women navigating perimenopause can aid their bodies in reducing inflammation levels and enhancing their overall health.

Transitioning through perimenopause following the anti-inflammatory diet can help alleviate symptoms and enhance the quality of life. Apart from choices, lifestyle elements like managing stress, engaging in activity, and getting adequate sleep play a role in inflammation. By addressing these aspects and making adjustments, women can better support their bodies in reducing inflammation and enhancing their well-being during perimenopause. Regular physical exercise incorporating stress-relieving practices such as meditation or yoga and prioritizing sleep contribute to lowering inflammation levels and fostering health.

Recognizing the impact of inflammation on health during perimenopause and taking measures to reduce it through changes and lifestyle modifications can aid women in navigating this life stage more smoothly with increased vitality. Embracing an anti-inflammatory diet and healthy lifestyle practices enables women to enhance their general health, alleviate symptoms, and optimize well-being during perimenopause.

The Influence of Hormones on Cardiac Wellness

Hormones play a role in women's health, particularly heart health. As women age, hormonal shifts can notably impact the system, heightening their vulnerability to heart disease. Recognizing how hormones influence well-being is vital for perimenopausal women striving to boost their health.

Estrogen – a hormone for women – has been found to benefit the heart by supporting healthy blood vessels, regulating cholesterol levels, and reducing inflammation. Nevertheless, as women near menopause, diminishing estrogen levels increase the risk of heart disease. Henceforth, it's imperative for women, in this phase, to be mindful of their equilibrium and take measures to promote heart wellness.

Progesterone, another hormone for women, also plays a role in maintaining heart health. It assists in regulating blood pressure and lowering the chances of blood clot formation. When progesterone levels are out of balance, issues like hypertension and increased clotting may arise, potentially contributing to heart conditions. By monitoring and ensuring progesterone levels, women can promote their heart health and lessen the likelihood of cardiovascular problems.

Cortisol, famously known as the stress hormone, also impacts heart health. Prolonged stress can elevate cortisol levels, leading to heightened blood pressure, cholesterol levels, and inflammation—all risk factors linked to heart disease. Women in perimenopause facing elevated stress levels should focus on managing stress and maintaining a cortisol balance to safeguard their heart health.

In summary, hormones play a role in midlife women's wellness. By comprehending how estrogen, progesterone, and cortisol influence heart health, women can take measures to maintain equilibrium and enhance their health. Addressing imbalances through lifestyle adjustments that support heart wellness can help women lower their risk of heart disease and improve their quality of life.

Typical Hormonal Imbalances Among Women

Hormones are indispensable for women's health and well-being as they age.

Hormonal imbalances can cause symptoms and health problems that affect not only physical health but also emotional and mental well-being. Let's talk about some imbalances women might face during menopause and how they can influence heart health and overall well-being.

A typical hormonal imbalance in women is thyroid dysfunction, hypothyroidism, where the thyroid gland doesn't produce thyroid hormone. Symptoms of hypothyroidism may include fatigue, weight gain, hair loss, and feelings of depression. Thyroid dysfunction could also affect heart health by raising the risk of cholesterol, hypertension, and heart disease.

Cortisol imbalance is another problem that can impact women during this life stage. Prolonged stress might disrupt the HPA axis, leading to cortisol levels that disturb hormone balance and influence heart health.

Cortisol imbalance may manifest as weight gain, trouble sleeping, feelings of anxiousness, and a weakened immune system. To balance cortisol levels and enhance well-being, it's important to manage stress by making lifestyle adjustments, practicing relaxation methods, and taking care of yourself properly.

As women age, insulin resistance can become an issue, especially for those leading a sedentary lifestyle with poor eating habits. When the body's cells resist insulin's effects, it results in blood sugar levels, increasing the chances of developing type 2 diabetes and heart problems. Controlling insulin resistance through diet, exercise, and weight management is vital for preventing heart-related complications and supporting health.

In summary, recognizing and addressing imbalances plays a role in sustaining optimal health for aging women. By understanding the indications of concerns like estrogen dominance, thyroid irregularities, cortisol imbalance, and insulin resistance, women can proactively work towards harmonizing their hormones to enhance heart health. Collaboration with healthcare professionals adopting lifestyle modifications and incorporating targeted interventions can assist women in this age bracket in achieving equilibrium while promoting cardiometabolic well-being over time.

Polycystic Ovary Syndrome (PCOS) stands out as a condition affecting women during their reproductive years.

Women with PCOS experience cycles, elevated levels of male hormones, and the presence of small cysts on their ovaries. While PCOS is commonly linked to fertility challenges, recent studies have highlighted the increased risk of heart disease in women with this condition. A key characteristic of PCOS is insulin resistance, which hampers the body's ability to utilize insulin effectively. Chronic inflammation often accompanies syndrome (PCOS), leading to a range of symptoms in affected individuals. This inflammation can result in heightened insulin levels in the bloodstream, elevating the risk of developing type 2 diabetes and heart disease. Research indicates that women with PCOS are at a risk—two to four times more—of developing heart disease compared to those without the condition.

Moreover, women with PCOS are predisposed to heart disease risk factors like hypertension, high cholesterol levels, and obesity. When combined with insulin resistance, these factors create an environment for heart disease progression. It is crucial for women with PCOS to take measures to manage their health and minimize their susceptibility to heart disease.

One practical approach for reducing the risk of heart disease among women with PCOS involves focusing on balance through lifestyle modifications.

Maintaining weight means eating a rounded diet rich in fruits, vegetables, and whole grains, and engaging in regular exercise is essential for overall health. These lifestyle adjustments can enhance insulin sensitivity, reduce inflammation, and decrease cholesterol levels, all of which contribute to reducing the risk of heart disease.

In addition to making lifestyle changes, women with PCOS can benefit from collaborating with healthcare providers to monitor their heart health and address any risk factors they may face. This may involve undergoing screenings for blood pressure, cholesterol, and blood sugar levels while addressing any concerns related to heart disease. By managing their health, women with PCOS can lower their risk of heart disease and enhance their general well-being.

Thyroid disorders impact the health of women in their childbearing years. The thyroid gland regulates metabolism and energy levels. When it malfunctions, it can lead to health complications, including issues. It is essential for women within this age group to understand the link between thyroid disorders and heart health so they can take measures to safeguard their well-being.

One prevalent thyroid disorder that affects heart health is hypothyroidism—a condition where the thyroid gland fails to produce thyroid hormones. Hypothyroidism could result in a heart rate, raised cholesterol levels, and an increased risk of heart disease.

Women who have hypothyroidism should collaborate closely with their healthcare provider to keep an eye on their thyroid levels and make any necessary changes to their medication to maintain heart health.

Hyperthyroidism, a condition in which the thyroid gland produces too much hormone, can also impact heart health. Women with hyperthyroidism might experience a fast heart rate, palpitations, and an elevated risk of fibrillation. It's crucial for women in this age bracket to be mindful of hyperthyroidism symptoms and seek treatment to manage their thyroid levels and safeguard their heart well-being.

Apart from thyroid issues, hormonal imbalances can also influence women's heart health. Estrogen and progesterone levels can affect cholesterol, blood pressure, and cardiovascular well-being. Women should collaborate with their healthcare providers to tackle imbalances and create a strategy to optimize hormone levels for heart health.

Women need to care for their health by working with healthcare providers to monitor thyroid levels, address imbalances, and safeguard cardiovascular health.

Understanding the link between thyroid issues, hormonal imbalances, and heart wellness enables women to empower themselves to manage their health and enhance their quality of life.

In conclusion, hormones play a significant role in heart health for midlife women. By understanding how hormones such as estrogen, progesterone, and cortisol impact heart health, women can take steps to support their hormonal balance and improve their overall well-being. By addressing hormone imbalances and making lifestyle changes to support heart health, women can reduce their risk of heart disease and improve their quality of life.

Polycystic Ovary Syndrome (PCOS) and Heart Disease Risk

Polycystic Ovary Syndrome (PCOS) is a disorder that affects women of reproductive age. It is known for causing periods, elevated hormone levels, and small cysts on the ovaries. While PCOS is often associated with fertility issues, recent studies suggest that women with PCOS face an increased risk of developing heart disease. This heightened risk is linked to insulin resistance, inflammation, and other factors commonly seen in individuals with PCOS. The combination of these factors can lead to insulin levels in the bloodstream, raising the likelihood of developing type 2 diabetes and heart disease. Research indicates that women diagnosed with PCOS are at a two to four times higher risk of heart disease compared to those without the condition. Moreover, women with PCOS are more prone to heart disease risk factors like high blood pressure, elevated cholesterol levels, and obesity. Managing these risk factors effectively is essential for women with PCOS to safeguard their health.

One key strategy to lessen the chances of heart disease in women with PCOS involves focusing on harmonizing hormones through lifestyle adjustments. This encompasses maintaining a healthy weight, consuming a rounded diet rich in fruits, vegetables, and whole grains, and engaging in regular physical activity. These lifestyle modifications can enhance insulin sensitivity, diminish inflammation, and decrease cholesterol levels, all contributing to reducing the risk of heart disease.

Alongside lifestyle alterations, women with PCOS could also collaborate with a healthcare provider to monitor their heart health and address any risk factors they may face. This may entail undergoing screenings for blood pressure, cholesterol, and blood sugar levels while openly discussing any concerns regarding heart disease. By taking a role in managing their health, women with PCOS can mitigate the risk of heart disease and enhance their overall well-being.

Thyroid Disorders and Heart Health

Thyroid disorders can significantly impact heart health for women of childbearing age. The thyroid gland plays a crucial role in regulating metabolism and energy levels. When it is not functioning correctly, it can lead to various health issues, including cardiovascular problems. Women in this age group must know the connection between thyroid disorders and heart health to ensure they take the necessary steps to protect their cardiovascular well-being.

One common thyroid disorder that can affect heart health is hypothyroidism, which occurs when the thyroid gland does not produce enough thyroid hormones. This can lead to a slow heart rate, increased cholesterol levels, and a higher risk of developing heart disease. Women with hypothyroidism should work closely with their healthcare provider to monitor their thyroid levels and make any necessary adjustments to their medication to keep their hearts healthy.

On the other hand, hyperthyroidism, where the thyroid gland produces too much thyroid hormone, can also impact heart health. Women with hyperthyroidism may experience a rapid heart rate, palpitations, and an increased risk of atrial fibrillation. Women in this age group need to be aware of the symptoms of hyperthyroidism and seek treatment to help manage their thyroid levels and protect their heart health.

In addition to thyroid disorders, hormonal imbalances can also play a role in heart health for women. Estrogen and progesterone levels can impact cholesterol, blood pressure, and cardiovascular health. Women need to work with their healthcare provider to address hormonal imbalances and develop a plan to optimize their hormone levels to support heart health.

Women must be proactive about their health and work with their healthcare provider to monitor their thyroid levels, address hormonal imbalances, and protect their cardiovascular well-being. By understanding the connection between thyroid disorders, hormonal imbalances, and heart health, women can empower themselves to take control of their health and improve their overall well-being.

How Inflammation Affects Metabolism in Perimenopause

Many women experience changes in their metabolism during perimenopause that can be attributed to the effects of inflammation on the body. Inflammation is a natural response by the immune system to protect the body from harmful stimuli, such as pathogens, injuries, or irritants. However, chronic inflammation can negatively affect metabolism, leading to weight gain, insulin resistance, and other metabolic issues.

One way inflammation affects metabolism in perimenopause is by disrupting the balance of hormones in the body. Inflammation can lead to imbalances in hormones such as insulin, cortisol, and estrogen, which play a crucial role in regulating metabolism. These hormone imbalances can make it harder for the body to regulate blood sugar levels, leading to insulin resistance and weight gain.

Additionally, inflammation can affect the function of mitochondria, the powerhouse of the cells responsible for producing energy. When inflammation disrupts mitochondrial function, it can decrease energy production and cause slower metabolism. This can make it harder for women in perimenopause to maintain a healthy weight and have enough energy to support their daily activities.

Furthermore, inflammation can also increase the production of free radicals in the body, which are unstable molecules that can damage cells and contribute to aging and disease. This oxidative stress caused by inflammation can further disrupt metabolism and lead to weight gain and other metabolic issues. By reducing inflammation through diet and lifestyle changes, women in perimenopause can support their metabolism and overall health.

To combat the effects of inflammation on metabolism in perimenopause, women can focus on following an anti-inflammatory diet that includes plenty of fruits, vegetables, lean proteins, and healthy fats. Additionally, incorporating regular exercise, stress management techniques, and adequate sleep can help reduce inflammation and support a healthy metabolism. By proactively managing inflammation, women can reset their metabolism and improve their overall health during the perimenopausal years.

Identifying Inflammatory Triggers in Perimenopause

Many women experience an increase in inflammatory symptoms such as bloating, joint pain, and fatigue during perimenopause. Identifying inflammation triggers can be crucial in managing these symptoms and improving overall health. In this subchapter, we will explore common inflammatory triggers in perimenopause and how to address them through dietary and lifestyle changes.

One of the primary inflammatory triggers in perimenopause is hormonal fluctuations. As estrogen levels decrease during this time, the body can experience increased inflammation. By balancing hormones through proper nutrition and lifestyle choices, women can help reduce inflammation and alleviate symptoms. Incorporating foods rich in phytoestrogens, such as flaxseeds and soy products, can help balance hormone levels and reduce inflammation.

Another common trigger of inflammation in perimenopause is stress. Chronic stress can lead to increased cortisol levels, a hormone that can trigger inflammation. Managing stress through relaxation techniques such as meditation, yoga, and deep breathing exercises can help reduce inflammation and improve overall health. Incorporating adaptogenic herbs such as ashwagandha and Rhodiola into your diet can help support the body's stress response and reduce inflammation.

Dietary factors can also significantly trigger inflammation in perimenopause. Foods high in sugar, refined carbohydrates, and trans fats can increase inflammation. By following a women's anti-inflammatory diet, which focuses on whole, nutrient-dense foods such as fruits, vegetables, lean proteins, and healthy fats, women can help reduce inflammation and support their overall health. Avoiding processed foods, alcohol, and caffeine can also help reduce inflammation and improve symptoms.

In addition to dietary changes, lifestyle factors such as lack of exercise and poor sleep can also contribute to inflammation in perimenopause. Regular physical activity, such as walking, yoga, or strength training, can help reduce inflammation and improve overall health. Getting adequate quality sleep each night is also crucial in managing inflammation and supporting hormonal balance. By addressing these lifestyle factors, women can help reduce inflammation and improve their overall health during perimenopause.

In conclusion, identifying and addressing inflammatory triggers in perimenopause is essential in managing symptoms and improving overall health. By balancing hormones, managing stress, following a women's anti-inflammatory diet, and incorporating regular exercise and quality sleep, women can help reduce inflammation and support their metabolic health during this transitional period. By making these changes, women can reset their health and improve their quality of life in perimenopause.

Chapter Three:

Developing a Diet Plan to Combat Inflammation

"There is no good food or bad food, the only truth that exists is food that helps the body be nourished. The Belev Method is about helping women identify their energy sources, via meals and snack times and finding a balance between them. The focus is to feel fulfilled, satisfied and knowing that we're winning at the game of life by the food choices we make."

The Basics of an Anti-Inflammatory Diet

This chapter will delve into the basics of an anti-inflammatory diet and how it can benefit perimenopausal women in resetting their health and managing symptoms associated with this stage of life. As women enter perimenopause, hormonal changes can lead to increased inflammation in the body, which can exacerbate symptoms such as hot flashes, mood swings, and weight gain. Focusing on an anti-inflammatory diet during this transitional period can help reduce inflammation and support their overall health and well-being.

The foundation of an anti-inflammatory diet is centered around whole, nutrient-dense foods rich in antioxidants and anti-inflammatory compounds. It includes many fruits and vegetables, whole grains, lean proteins, and healthy fats such as avocado, nuts, and olive oil. By incorporating these foods into your daily meals, you can help reduce inflammation in the body and support a healthy metabolism, which is crucial for managing weight and energy levels during perimenopause.

In addition to focusing on specific foods, an anti-inflammatory diet also involves minimizing or eliminating processed foods, refined sugars, and unhealthy fats that can contribute to inflammation in the body. This means avoiding foods such as sugary snacks, fried foods, and processed meats, which can promote inflammation and worsen symptoms of perimenopause. By making conscious choices to limit these foods and focus on whole, nutrient-dense options, women can support their health and well-being during this stage of life.

Another critical aspect of an anti-inflammatory diet is staying hydrated and reducing alcohol consumption. Dehydration can exacerbate inflammation, so drinking plenty of water daily is essential to keep hydrated. Additionally, alcohol can increase inflammation and disrupt hormone balance, so it's best to limit consumption or avoid it altogether during perimenopause. By prioritizing hydration and reducing alcohol intake, women can support their bodies in managing inflammation and promoting overall health.

Overall, an anti-inflammatory diet can be a powerful tool for perimenopausal women looking to reset their health and manage symptoms associated with this stage of life. By focusing on whole, nutrient-dense foods, minimizing processed and inflammatory foods, and staying hydrated, women can support their bodies in reducing inflammation, balancing hormones, and promoting overall well-being during this transitional period. By making simple yet effective changes to their diet, women can take control of their health and thrive during perimenopause.

Foods to Include in Your Diet

As a perimenopausal woman, it is crucial to pay attention to the foods you include in your diet to support your health and well-being during this transitional phase of life. Choosing the right foods can help balance your hormones, reduce inflammation, and support your metabolism. This chapter will explore some essential foods to include in your diet to help you easily navigate perimenopause.

One of the most essential foods during perimenopause is leafy green vegetables. These nutrient-dense foods contain vitamins, minerals, and antioxidants that can support your overall health. Leafy greens like spinach, kale, and collard greens are also high in fiber, which can help regulate your digestion and support a healthy metabolism. Try to incorporate a variety of leafy greens into your meals each day to reap the benefits.

Lean proteins are another essential food group to include during perimenopause. Protein is necessary to maintain muscle mass, support hormone production, and keep you full and satisfied. Opt for lean protein sources like chicken, fish, tofu, and legumes to support your metabolism and keep your energy levels stable throughout the day. Aim to include a source of protein in each meal to help balance your blood sugar and support your overall health.

In addition to leafy greens and lean proteins, it is essential to include healthy fats in your diet during perimenopause. Healthy fats, such as avocados, nuts, seeds, and olive oil, can help support hormone production, reduce inflammation, and support a healthy metabolism. Including various healthy fats in your diet can also help keep you full and satisfied, reducing the risk of overeating or cravings. Be sure to include a source of healthy fats in each meal to support your overall health during perimenopause.

In conclusion, nutrient-dense foods like leafy greens, lean proteins, and healthy fats during perimenopause can help support your health and well-being during this transitional phase. By focusing on whole, unprocessed foods and avoiding inflammatory foods like sugar and processed grains, you can easily support your metabolism, balance your hormones, and navigate perimenopause. Experiment with different foods and recipes to find what works best for your body, and remember to listen to your body's cues to determine what foods support your health and well-being during this time.

Foods to Avoid in Perimenopause

This subchapter will discuss the importance of being mindful of the foods you consume during perimenopause. Certain foods can exacerbate symptoms and make the transition more difficult as your body goes through hormonal changes. By avoiding these foods, you can better manage your symptoms and support your overall health during this stage of life.

One type of food to avoid during perimenopause is processed foods. These foods are often high in unhealthy fats, sugars, and preservatives, which can contribute to inflammation in the body. Inflammation can worsen symptoms such as hot flashes, mood swings, and weight gain. Cutting processed foods from your diet can reduce inflammation and support your body's natural detoxification processes.

Another food group to avoid during perimenopause is refined carbohydrates. Foods like white bread, pasta, and pastries can cause spikes in blood sugar levels, leading to energy crashes and weight gain. These foods can also disrupt hormone balance and contribute to insulin resistance, which can make perimenopausal symptoms more severe. Instead, focus on whole grains like quinoa, brown rice, and oats, which provide sustained energy and support healthy hormone levels.

Dairy products are another food group to consider avoiding during perimenopause. Dairy can be inflammatory for some individuals, particularly those with lactose intolerance or sensitivities to dairy proteins. Inflammation can worsen symptoms like bloating, joint pain, and skin issues. Consider alternatives like almond or coconut milk, dairy-free yogurts, and plant-based cheeses to support your digestive health and reduce inflammation during perimenopause.

Lastly, it's essential to be mindful of caffeine and alcohol consumption during perimenopause. Both substances can disrupt hormone balance and exacerbate symptoms like hot flashes, insomnia, and mood swings. Caffeine can also contribute to anxiety and irritability, while alcohol can disrupt sleep patterns and contribute to weight gain. Limiting your intake of these substances can help you better manage your symptoms and support your overall health during perimenopause.

Avoiding these foods during perimenopause can support your body's natural detoxification processes, reduce inflammation, and manage your symptoms more effectively. Everyone's body is different, so listening to your body and making choices supporting your health needs is essential. With a focus on whole, nutrient-dense foods and mindful eating habits, you can navigate perimenopause gracefully and efficiently.

Breakfast Ideas for Hormone Balance

Breakfast is often touted as the most important meal of the day, and for good reason. Regarding hormone balance, what you eat for breakfast can make a big difference in how your hormones function throughout the day; for women of childbearing age who want to improve their hormone balance and heart health, starting the day with the right breakfast choices is critical.

A smoothie with hormone-balancing ingredients such as flaxseeds, spinach, and berries is an excellent breakfast for hormone balance. Flaxseeds are rich in omega-3 fatty acids, which can help support hormone production and reduce inflammation. Spinach is loaded with nutrients like iron and Magnesium, which are essential for hormone balance. Berries are high in antioxidants, which can help protect your cells from damage and support overall hormone health.

Another breakfast option for hormone balance is a bowl of overnight oats topped with hormone-balancing nuts and seeds like almonds, walnuts, and chia seeds. Oats are a great source of fiber, which can help regulate blood sugar levels and support hormone balance. Nuts and seeds are rich in healthy fats and protein, essential for hormone production and overall health. Adding a sprinkle of cinnamon can also help balance blood sugar levels and support hormone function.

A breakfast of avocado toast with eggs can be an excellent option for women looking to support their hormone balance and heart health. Avocados are rich in healthy fats and fiber, which can help support hormone production and regulate blood sugar levels. Eggs are a great source of protein and nutrients like choline, essential for hormone balance and heart health. Adding a sprinkle of turmeric to your eggs can also help reduce inflammation and support hormone function.

Lunch and Dinner Recipes for Heart Health

We will explore some delicious and heart-healthy lunch and dinner recipes. These recipes are designed to help balance hormones and improve heart health for women in perimenopause. Incorporating these nutrient-dense meals into your diet can support your overall well-being and reduce your risk of heart disease.

For lunch, try a Mediterranean-inspired quinoa salad. This dish contains heart-healthy ingredients like olive oil, tomatoes, cucumbers, and feta cheese. Quinoa is an excellent source of protein and fiber, which can help regulate hormones and support cardiovascular health. To make this salad even more nutritious, add some grilled chicken or chickpeas for an extra protein boost.

Another delicious lunch option is a salmon avocado wrap. Salmon is rich in omega-3 fatty acids, which have been shown to reduce inflammation and improve heart health. Avocado is also a great source of healthy fats and fiber, making this wrap a nutrient-dense and satisfying meal. Serve it with mixed greens or a cup of vegetable soup for a complete and balanced lunch.

For dinner, consider making a hearty lentil and vegetable stew. Lentils are high in fiber and protein, making them an excellent choice for hormone balance and heart health. This stew is also packed with colorful vegetables like carrots, bell peppers, and spinach, which provide essential vitamins and

Incorporating these lunch and dinner recipes into your weekly meal plan can help you maintain hormonal balance and support your heart health as a woman in the perimenopausal age group. You can nourish your body and reduce your risk of chronic diseases like heart disease by choosing nutrient-dense ingredients like salmon, quinoa, lentils, and vegetables. Experiment with different flavors and ingredients to find recipes that you enjoy and that make you feel your best. Food is medicine; choosing the right ingredients can support your hormones and heart for optimal health and well-being.

Snack Options for Hormonal Imbalance

Snacking can be tricky, especially when balancing hormones and improving heart health. Women often struggle with hormonal imbalances that can affect their overall well-being. However, choosing the right snacks can make a big difference in managing these imbalances, supporting your heart health, and exploring snack options that can help you regain hormonal balance and improve your heart health.

Nuts and seeds are a great snack for women dealing with hormonal imbalances. These nutrient-dense snacks are packed with healthy fats, protein, and fiber, which can help stabilize blood sugar levels and support hormone production. Almonds, walnuts, chia seeds, and flaxseeds are all excellent choices for women looking to balance their hormones and improve heart health. Nuts and seeds are a great snack for women dealing with hormonal imbalances. These nutrient-dense snacks are packed with healthy fats, protein, and fiber, which can help stabilize blood sugar levels and support hormone production. Almonds, walnuts, chia seeds, and flaxseeds are all excellent choices for women looking to balance their hormones and improve heart health.

Another fantastic snack option is Greek yogurt. This creamy and delicious snack is rich in protein and probiotics, which can help support gut health and hormone balance. Probiotics have been shown to regulate hormones, so incorporating Greek yogurt into your snacking routine can be a great way to support your hormonal health.

Avocado toast is a delicious and nutritious snack for women looking to balance their hormones and improve heart health. Avocados are rich in monounsaturated fats, which can help lower harmful cholesterol levels and support heart health. Pairing avocado with whole-grain toast can provide a satisfying and filling snack to help stabilize blood sugar levels and support hormone balance.

In addition to these snack options, incorporating fruits and vegetables into your snacking routine can help support hormonal balance and heart health. Berries, apples, carrots, and bell peppers are all excellent choices for women looking to balance their hormones and improve their heart health. These nutrient-dense snacks are packed with vitamins, minerals, and antioxidants that can help support overall well-being and hormone balance.

Women can support their hormonal balance and improve their heart health by choosing nutrient-dense snacks like nuts and seeds, Greek yogurt, avocado toast, and fruits and vegetables. These delicious and satisfying snack options provide essential nutrients that can help women on their journey to hormonal balance and improved cardiometabolic health.

Chapter Four:

Making Lifestyle Adjustments for Better Metabolic Functioning

"Counseling women to make lifestyle changes is one of the most important pieces of advice. To be able to teach the art of habit stacking in order to bio hack one's lifestyle into a fat burning lean muscle building machine is the goal for the Belev method. Our body has the ability to rejuvenate itself on a daily basis. The key is in all the micro decisions we make for the macro perspective of life. That is if you're hoping for a life expectancy of 100 years of age."

The Importance of Exercise in Perimenopause

Perimenopause is a time of significant hormonal changes in a woman's body, which can lead to a variety of symptoms such as hot flashes, mood swings, and weight gain. Regular exercise is one of the most effective ways to manage these symptoms and support overall health. Exercise is crucial in balancing hormones, reducing inflammation, and supporting metabolic health, making it an essential component of any perimenopausal women's wellness routine.

Regular physical activity has been shown to help regulate hormone levels during perimenopause, particularly estrogen and progesterone. These hormones play a vital role in the menstrual cycle and can become imbalanced during perimenopause, leading to symptoms such as irregular periods and mood swings. Exercise can help regulate these hormone levels, reducing the severity of these symptoms and promoting overall hormonal balance.

In addition to hormone regulation, exercise is also essential for reducing inflammation. Inflammation is a crucial driver of many chronic health conditions, including heart disease, diabetes, and arthritis, and can be exacerbated during perimenopause. Regular exercise helps to reduce inflammation by decreasing levels of pro-inflammatory molecules in the body, leading to improved overall health and reduced risk of chronic disease.

Furthermore, exercise plays a crucial role in supporting metabolic health during perimenopause. As women age, their metabolism naturally slows down, making it easier to gain weight and more challenging to lose. Regular exercise helps to rev up the metabolism, burn calories and fat more efficiently, and support weight management. Additionally, exercise can help improve insulin sensitivity, reducing the risk of developing insulin resistance and type 2 diabetes, which are common concerns for perimenopausal women.

Incorporating regular exercise into your daily routine is essential for supporting your health and well-being during perimenopause. Whether it's through yoga, strength training, or cardio workouts, finding an exercise routine you enjoy and can stick to is critical. By balancing hormones, reducing inflammation, and supporting metabolic health, exercise can help you navigate the challenges of perimenopause with grace and vitality.

Stress Management Techniques for Metabolic Health

Stress management techniques can help improve metabolic health in perimenopausal women. As we age and undergo hormonal changes, stress can significantly impact our metabolism and overall health. By practicing these techniques, you can better manage stress levels and support your body's metabolic functions.

One effective stress management technique for perimenopausal women is mindfulness meditation. This practice involves focusing on the present moment and being aware of your thoughts and feelings without judgment. Studies have shown that regular meditation can reduce stress hormones, improve insulin sensitivity, and promote weight loss. Consider incorporating a daily meditation into your routine to help manage stress and support your metabolic health.

Another helpful technique for managing stress is deep breathing exercises. When we are stressed, our breathing tends to become shallow and rapid, which can further exacerbate feelings of anxiety and tension. By practicing deep breathing exercises, you can activate the body's relaxation response, lower cortisol levels, and promote better digestion and metabolism. Take a few minutes daily to focus on your breath and engage in deep, slow inhales and exhales to calm your mind and body.

Physical activity is also crucial for managing stress and supporting metabolic health. Exercise has been shown to reduce stress hormones, improve insulin sensitivity, and boost metabolism. Aim to incorporate cardiovascular, strength training, and flexibility exercises into your routine to help manage stress levels and support your body's metabolic functions. Whether it's going for a walk, taking a yoga class, or hitting the gym, find activities that you enjoy and that make you feel good.

In addition to these techniques, it's important to prioritize self-care practices such as getting enough sleep, eating a balanced diet, and staying hydrated. Adequate rest, nutrition, and hydration are essential for managing stress and supporting metabolic health in perimenopausal women. Make sure to prioritize your well-being by getting enough sleep, eating various nutrient-dense foods, and drinking plenty of water throughout the day. Taking care of yourself and practicing these stress management techniques can support your body's metabolic functions and improve your overall health during perimenopause.

Sleep Strategies for Balancing Hormones and Metabolism

In the journey through perimenopause, one of the most crucial yet often overlooked aspects of health is the role of sleep in balancing hormones and metabolism. As women in this stage of life experience fluctuations in hormone levels, proper sleep becomes increasingly crucial for overall well-being. This subchapter will explore various sleep strategies to help perimenopausal women optimize their hormone levels and support their metabolism.

One key strategy for improving sleep quality is establishing a regular sleep routine. Going to bed and waking up at the same time each day can help regulate the body's internal clock, making it easier to fall asleep and stay asleep throughout the night. Creating a calming bedtime routine, such as taking a warm bath or practicing relaxation techniques, can signal to the body that it is time to wind down and prepare for sleep.

Another critical factor in balancing hormones and metabolism through sleep is creating a sleep-friendly environment. This includes keeping the bedroom dark, calm, and quiet and investing in comfortable mattresses and pillows. Limiting exposure to screens and electronic devices before bed can also improve sleep quality, as the blue light emitted by these devices can disrupt the body's production of melatonin, a hormone that regulates sleep-wake cycles.

In addition to establishing a regular sleep routine and creating a sleep-friendly environment, incorporating relaxation practices such as meditation, deep breathing, or gentle yoga before bed can help calm the mind and body, making it easier to fall asleep. Stress management techniques, such as journaling or counseling, can also be beneficial for improving sleep quality and supporting hormone balance during perimenopause.

Finally, incorporating a healthy diet and regular physical activity into your daily routine can support hormone balance and metabolism, improving sleep quality. Foods rich in Magnesium, zinc, and B vitamins can help regulate hormone levels and support the body's natural sleep-wake cycle. Regular exercise, such as walking, yoga, or strength training, can also help improve sleep quality and overall health during perimenopause. Perimenopausal women can support their hormone balance and metabolism by implementing these sleep strategies and prioritizing rest, improving their health and well-being during this transitional stage.

Chapter Five:

Exploring Supplements and
Herbal Remedies for Supporting Metabolism

have witnessed many miraculous changes to the human body once it's given the appropriate nutrition and similarly, herbs and supplements provide the body with healing. I prefer not to use the term alternative healing because it is counterintuitive, I would rather refer to healing with herbs and supplements as the truth in healing."

- Isabel Bogdan

Essential Supplements for Perimenopausal Women

As women enter perimenopause, their bodies undergo significant hormonal changes that can lead to a variety of symptoms, including hot flashes, mood swings, and weight gain. Perimenopausal women must prioritize their nutrition and supplement intake to help manage these symptoms and support overall health during this transitional period.

One essential supplement for perimenopausal women is Magnesium. Magnesium plays a crucial role in over 300 enzymatic reactions in the body, including those involved in energy production and muscle function. Many women in perimenopause are deficient in Magnesium, which can contribute to symptoms such as muscle cramps, fatigue, and insomnia. By supplementing with Magnesium, women can support their overall health and well-being during this time of transition. While there are different types of Magnesium, for clarity, we will be focusing on the benefits of Magnesium Glycinate and an initial dose of 100mg daily an hour before bed.

Another essential supplement for perimenopausal women is vitamin D. Vitamin D is necessary for bone health, immune function, and mood regulation. Many women in perimenopause are deficient in vitamin D due to decreased sun exposure and changes in hormone levels. By supplementing with vitamin D, women can support their bone health and overall immune function and improve their mood during this challenging time. The initial dose of Vitamin D should be 2000iu once daily.

In addition to magnesium and vitamin D, perimenopausal women may benefit from supplementing with omega-3 fatty acids. Omega-3 fatty acids are essential for brain and heart health and for reducing inflammation in the body. Many women in perimenopause experience increased inflammation due to hormonal changes, which can contribute to symptoms such as joint pain, bloating, and mood swings. By supplementing with omega-3 fatty acids, women can support their overall health and reduce inflammation with an initial dose of 1000 mg once daily.

Furthermore, perimenopausal women may also consider supplementing with probiotics to support their gut health. The gut microbiome is crucial in immune function, digestion, and mood regulation. Many women in perimenopause experience change in their gut health due to hormonal fluctuations and stress. By supplementing with probiotics, women can support their gut health and overall well-being during this challenging time.

In conclusion, perimenopausal women can benefit from supplementing with critical nutrients such as Magnesium, vitamin D, omega-3 fatty acids, and probiotics to support their overall health and well-being during this transitional period. By prioritizing their nutrition and supplement intake, women can better manage symptoms such as hot flashes, mood swings, and weight gain and support their long-term health as they navigate perimenopause.

Herbs for Hormone Balance and Metabolic Health

In the journey through perimenopause, many women experience hormonal imbalances that can impact their overall health and well-being. One way to support hormone balance and metabolic health during this time is through herbs. Herbs have been used for centuries to help regulate hormones and support the body's natural metabolic processes. This subchapter will explore some top herbs to help you reach metabolic mastery.

One powerful herb for hormone balance is maca root. Maca is a Peruvian plant used for centuries to support hormonal health in both men and women. It is known for regulating the endocrine system and supporting healthy hormone production. Maca can be taken in supplement form or added to smoothies and other recipes for an easy way to incorporate it into your daily routine.

Another herb that can support hormone balance and metabolic health is ashwagandha. Ashwagandha is an adaptogen herb that helps the body adapt to stress and balance hormone levels. It benefits women experiencing adrenal fatigue and high cortisol levels, which can impact hormone balance. Ashwagandha can be taken in supplement form or brewed into a calming tea to help support your body's natural healing processes.

Turmeric is another powerful herb for hormone balance and metabolic health. It contains curcumin, a compound with anti-inflammatory and antioxidant properties. These properties can help reduce inflammation, often a factor in hormonal imbalances and metabolic issues. Turmeric can be added to soups, stews, and other recipes to help support your body's natural detoxification processes and promote overall health.

Many other natural remedies can support hormone balance and metabolic health during perimenopause. Herbs like holy basil, rhodiola, and licorice root can also benefit women looking to reset their health and support their bodies during this transition. Incorporating these herbs into your daily routine can help support your body's natural healing processes and promote overall well-being.

Overall, herbs can be a valuable tool for women looking to balance their hormones and support their metabolic health during perimenopause. By incorporating these herbs into your daily routine and working with a knowledgeable healthcare provider, you can help reset your health and support your body's natural healing processes during this critical time of transition.

How to Safely Incorporate Supplements and Herbs into Your Routine

Incorporating supplements and herbs into your routine can be a great way to support your health during perimenopause. However, it's essential to approach this cautiously and ensure That goals for metabolic mastery are set for reclaiming your health during perimenopause. As women in this stage of life, our bodies undergo significant changes that can impact our metabolism and overall well-being. By setting clear and achievable goals, we can take control of our health and work towards resetting our metabolism for optimal health.

Establishing a healthy eating plan is one of the first goals to consider when embarking on a metabolic reset journey. Our bodies may become more sensitive to certain foods in perimenopause, leading to inflammation and metabolic imbalances. Following a women's anti-inflammatory diet can help our bodies reduce inflammation and promote optimal metabolic function. Setting a goal to plan and prep healthy, nourishing meals can help us stay on track and fuel our bodies with the nutrients they need to thrive.

Another essential goal for metabolic mastery is incorporating regular physical activity into our daily routine. Exercise benefits our physical health and is crucial in boosting our metabolism and managing weight during perimenopause. Setting a goal to move our bodies regularly, whether through strength training, yoga, or walking, can help us maintain a healthy weight and support our metabolic function. By setting achievable exercise goals, we can prioritize our health and well-being during this transformative stage of life.

In addition to diet and exercise, setting goals for stress management is essential for metabolic mastery in perimenopause. Chronic stress can negatively impact our metabolism and overall health, leading to weight gain and inflammation. By setting goals to prioritize self-care activities such as meditation, mindfulness, or journaling, we can reduce stress levels and support our bodies in achieving metabolic balance. Taking time for ourselves and practicing self-care can profoundly impact our health and well-being during perimenopause.

Lastly, setting goals for metabolic mastery also involves tracking our progress and making adjustments as needed. By setting measurable objectives, such as weight loss or improved energy levels, we can monitor our progress and change our diet, exercise, and stress management strategies accordingly. Keeping a journal or using a tracking app can help us stay accountable and motivated on our metabolic reset journey. By setting clear and achievable goals, we can empower ourselves to take control of our health and achieve metabolic mastery during perimenopause.

Monitoring Your Symptoms and Progress

As you embark on your journey to reset your health in perimenopause, it is crucial to monitor your symptoms and progress along the way closely. Keeping track of how you feel physically and emotionally can provide valuable insights into how your body responds to the changes you are making. By paying attention to your symptoms, you can adjust your diet and lifestyle to support your overall health and well-being better.

One way to monitor your symptoms is to keep a journal to track your energy levels, mood, sleep quality, and any physical symptoms you may be experiencing. Tracking can help you identify patterns and triggers that may impact your health. For example, if you feel more fatigued after eating certain foods, consider eliminating them from your diet to see if your symptoms improve.

In addition to keeping a symptom journal, tracking your progress toward your health goals is essential. A journal can be a tool for monitoring your weight, body measurements, and any changes in your lab results. By regularly checking in on your progress, you can celebrate the positive changes you are making and stay motivated to continue on your journey to better health.

Another helpful tool for monitoring your symptoms and progress is working with a healthcare provider specializing in women's health and metabolic issues. They can help you interpret your symptoms and lab results and guide your diet and lifestyle. A knowledgeable healthcare provider on your team can help ensure you are on the right track to achieving your health goals.

Remember, each woman's journey through perimenopause is unique, and what works for one person may not work for another. By monitoring your symptoms and progress, you can tailor your approach to resetting your health to best suit your needs. Stay committed to taking care of yourself, and with time and dedication, you can achieve optimal health and well-being during this transformative phase of life.

Making Adjustments to Your Diet and Lifestyle Plan

First and foremost, it's essential to consult with a healthcare provider before starting any new supplement or herb regimen. They can help you determine which supplements are safe for you and any potential interactions with medications you may be taking. Your healthcare provider can also help you choose the proper dosage for each supplement, as taking too much can negatively affect your health.

When choosing supplements and herbs, it's essential to do your research and select high-quality products from reputable sources. Look for supplements that have been tested for purity and potency, and choose organic herbs that are free from contaminants. It's also a good idea to look for supplements specifically formulated for women in perimenopause, as they may contain ingredients tailored to your unique needs during this time of life.

When incorporating supplements and herbs into your routine, it's essential to start with one regimen at a time and monitor how your body reacts. Pay attention to any changes in your symptoms or overall well-being, and adjust your regimen accordingly. It's also a good idea to keep a journal to track your progress and note any changes you experience.

In conclusion, incorporating supplements and herbs into your routine can be a helpful way to support your health during perimenopause. You can safely incorporate supplements and herbs into your daily routine by consulting with a healthcare provider, choosing high-quality products, starting slowly, and monitoring your progress. Remember to listen to your body and make adjustments to ensure you benefit most from your supplement regimen.

Chapter Six:

Monitoring Your Journey and Tweaking Your Strategy

"Every week I would ask the patients to bring me their food diary, in it was written down the times and types of food they ate, then a number that would describe their glucose level. There was indeed a direct relationship with the number and the meal, the intention of having the patient write everything down was to be able to educate the patient and teach them exactly what it was that needed to change, you see we all need goals. What would you say are your goals?"

Setting Goals for Metabolic Mastery

Women in the perimenopause stage of life experience significant hormonal changes that can affect their metabolism, energy levels, and overall health. However, by taking charge of our diet and lifestyle, we can support our bodies during this transition period. This proactive approach can promote optimal health and well-being, empowering us to manage perimenopause effectively.

One critical adjustment to consider is adopting an anti-inflammatory diet. Inflammation is a common factor in many chronic health conditions, including those that can be exacerbated during perimenopause, such as weight gain, fatigue, and mood swings. By focusing on whole, nutrient-dense foods that help reduce inflammation, we can support our metabolism and overall health. This may include incorporating more fruits and vegetables, healthy fats, and lean proteins into our meals while reducing our intake of processed foods, sugar, and refined carbohydrates.

Another critical aspect of managing perimenopause symptoms is maintaining a stable blood sugar level. Fluctuations in blood sugar can contribute to mood swings, fatigue, and weight gain, common complaints during this stage of life. Regular, balanced meals and snacks that combine protein, healthy fats, and complex carbohydrates can help stabilize blood sugar levels and reduce these symptoms. Staying hydrated and regular exercise can also support healthy blood sugar regulation. Another option is wearing a continuous glucose monitor for 14 days to obtain data and understand diet and lifestyle trends. Wearing a glucometer will help you understand the fluctuations of blood sugar and your body's response to certain foods, activities, and lifestyle. This knowledge is powerful to integrate into an effective weight loss management program.

In addition to dietary changes, lifestyle adjustments can also play a significant role in managing perimenopause symptoms. Stress management techniques, such as mindfulness meditation, yoga, or deep breathing exercises, can help reduce the impact of stress on our bodies and support hormonal balance. Adequate sleep is also crucial, as poor sleep can exacerbate symptoms such as fatigue, mood swings, and weight gain. We can help our overall health and well-being during perimenopause by prioritizing healthy sleep habits, such as establishing a regular bedtime routine and creating a restful sleep environment.

Overall, making adjustments to your diet and lifestyle plan can have a significant impact on your experience of perimenopause. By focusing on an anti-inflammatory diet, stable blood sugar levels, stress management, and healthy sleep habits, you can support your metabolism, energy levels, and overall health during this transition period. Remember that every woman's experience of perimenopause is unique, so it may take some trial and error to find the strategies that work best for you. With patience and persistence, you can navigate this stage of life with grace and ease.

Chapter Seven:

Sustaining Metabolic Wellness Post Perimenopause

"Long term rejuvenation, this is the name of the game to the Belev method. To slow down the inflammaging process and help women learn to habit stack in order to bio-hack and live longer, richer, more balanced lives, for themselves and their families."

Long-Term Strategies for Metabolic Mastery

In this subchapter, we will delve into the long-term strategies that can help perimenopausal women achieve metabolic mastery and reset their health for the long haul. These strategies are essential for maintaining a healthy metabolism, managing weight, and reducing inflammation. Incorporating these strategies into your daily routine can optimize your health and well-being during this transitional phase.

One critical long-term strategy for metabolic mastery is adopting a women's anti-inflammatory diet. This diet focuses on reducing inflammation by incorporating foods rich in antioxidants, vitamins, and minerals. By eating a variety of colorful fruits and vegetables, lean proteins, healthy fats, and whole grains, you can help support your metabolism and overall health. This diet can also help regulate blood sugar levels, reduce cravings, and support hormonal balance during perimenopause.

In addition to following a women's anti-inflammatory diet, incorporating regular exercise into your routine is another essential long-term strategy for metabolic mastery. Exercise not only helps burn calories and support weight management, but it also helps reduce inflammation in the body, improve insulin sensitivity, and support cardiovascular health. Incorporating cardiovascular exercise, strength training, and flexibility exercises into your routine can help support your metabolism and overall health during perimenopause.

Another critical long-term strategy for metabolic mastery is managing stress and getting adequate sleep. Chronic stress and lack of sleep can harm your metabolism, hormone balance, and overall health. By incorporating stress-reducing activities such as meditation, yoga, and deep breathing exercises and getting at least 7-8 hours of quality sleep each night, you can help support your metabolism and overall well-being during perimenopause.

Finally, staying hydrated, managing portion sizes, and practicing mindful eating are other long-term strategies for metabolic mastery. Drinking an adequate amount of water each day can help support digestion, metabolism, and overall health. Managing portion sizes and practicing mindful eating can help you tune into your body's hunger and fullness cues, prevent overeating, and support weight management. By incorporating these long-term strategies into your daily routine, you can achieve metabolic mastery and reset your health during perimenopause.

Tips for Preventing Metabolic Issues in Menopause and Beyond

As women enter perimenopause and beyond, they may experience changes in their metabolism that can lead to weight gain, fatigue, and other health issues. Women need to take proactive steps to prevent metabolic problems during this stage of life. Here are some tips for avoiding metabolic issues in menopause and beyond.

First and foremost, it is essential to maintain a healthy diet rich in anti-inflammatory foods. This includes many fruits, vegetables, whole grains, and healthy fats like olive oil and avocado.

Avoiding processed foods, sugary drinks, and excessive red meat can help reduce inflammation and support a healthy metabolism.

Regular exercise is also crucial for preventing metabolic issues in menopause and beyond. Most days of the week, aim for at least 30 minutes of moderate exercise, such as brisk walking, cycling, or swimming. Strength training exercises can also help build muscle mass, boost metabolism, and prevent weight gain.

Stress management is another critical factor in preventing metabolic issues during menopause. Chronic stress can lead to hormonal imbalances that disrupt metabolism and contribute to weight gain. Practices like yoga, meditation, deep breathing exercises, and time in nature can help reduce stress and support a healthy metabolism.

Adequate sleep is also essential for preventing metabolic issues in menopause and beyond. Aim for seven to nine hours of quality sleep each night to support hormone regulation, reduce inflammation, and promote overall health. Poor sleep can disrupt metabolism and increase the risk of weight gain and other health issues.

Finally, working with a healthcare provider or nutritionist specializing in women's health and metabolic issues can provide personalized guidance and support for preventing metabolic issues during menopause and beyond. They can help create a customized diet and exercise plan, recommend supplements or medications, and monitor progress to ensure optimal health and well-being. By following these tips, perimenopausal women can take control of their metabolic health and prevent issues as they navigate this stage of life.

Celebrating Your Health and Wellness Achievements

Celebrating your health and wellness achievements is crucial to resetting your metabolic health as a perimenopausal woman. It's important to acknowledge and applaud yourself for your progress in taking control of your health during this transformative stage of life. By recognizing and celebrating your achievements, you are reinforcing positive behaviors and mindset shifts that will help you continue on your path to better health.

One way to celebrate your health and wellness achievements is by setting small, achievable goals for yourself. Whether committing to a daily walk, incorporating more vegetables into your meals, or practicing mindfulness and stress-reducing techniques, each small step towards better health is worth celebrating. By breaking down your goals into manageable tasks, you can track your progress and celebrate each milestone you reach.

Another way to celebrate your health and wellness achievements is to reward yourself for reaching your goals. After a week of consistently meeting your health and wellness goals, treat yourself to a massage, a new workout outfit, or a relaxing bath. By rewarding yourself, you reinforce the positive behaviors that have led to your success and motivate yourself to continue your journey toward better health.

Celebrating your health and wellness achievements also means acknowledging the obstacles you've overcome. Whether you overcome cravings for unhealthy foods, find the time to exercise amidst a busy schedule, or manage stress and emotional eating triggers, each obstacle you conquer is a reason to celebrate. By recognizing your resilience and determination, you can boost your confidence and motivation to continue making positive changes for your health.

In conclusion, celebrating your health and wellness achievements is an essential part of your journey to reset your metabolic health in perimenopause. By setting small, achievable goals, rewarding yourself for reaching milestones, and acknowledging the obstacles you've overcome, you can stay motivated and committed to improving your health. Remember to celebrate every step you take towards better health, as each achievement brings you closer to your ultimate goal of optimal health and wellness.

Hormone Balance and Heart Health Success Stories

Real-Life Testimonials of Hormone Balance Improvements

Let's explore real-life testimonials from women who have experienced significant improvements in their hormone balance through the strategies outlined in this book. These testimonials are potent examples of the transformative effects of balancing hormones on overall health and well-being.

One woman, Stacy, age 42, struggled with hormonal imbalances for years, experiencing symptoms such as mood swings, fatigue, and weight gain. After implementing the hormone-balancing diet and lifestyle changes recommended in this book, Stacy noticed a dramatic improvement in her symptoms. Her mood stabilized, her energy levels increased, and she was able to lose the excess weight that had been plaguing her for years. Stacy's story is a testament to the power of balancing hormones for overall health.

Another woman, Norah, age 38, suffered from irregular menstrual cycles and debilitating PMS symptoms for most of her adult life; every menstrual period was a difficult feat. Through the hormone-balancing protocols assisted by DNA testing, Emily was able to regulate her cycles and alleviate her PMS symptoms. She no longer experienced the intense mood swings and cramps that had previously disrupted her life every month. Emily's story demonstrates how balancing hormones can lead to a significant improvement in women's reproductive health.

A third testimonial comes from Lisa, age 45, who had been struggling with symptoms of perimenopause and flu-like symptoms prior to her menstrual cycle for several years. Hot flashes, night sweats, and insomnia were taking a toll on her physical and emotional well-being. After DNA testing we identified her histamine response was markedly causing the majority of her symptoms, by following the hormone-balancing recommendations in this book and introducing a low histamine lifestyle, Lisa experienced a reduction in her perimenopausal symptoms. Her hot flashes and flu-like symptoms became less frequent, her night sweats decreased, and she was able to get a restful night's sleep. Lisa's journey highlights the importance of hormone balance in managing the symptoms of perimenopause.

These real-life testimonials are just a few examples of the many women who have successfully improved their hormone balance and overall health through the strategies outlined in this book. By taking a proactive approach to hormone balance, women can experience significant improvements in their cardiometabolic health, reproductive health, and overall well-being. The stories of Stacy, Norah, and Lisa inspire women seeking to achieve optimal hormone balance and improve their heart health.

Heart Health Transformations Through Hormone Regulation

Heart health is a critical aspect of overall well-being, especially for women in perimenopause. Hormone regulation is crucial in maintaining a healthy heart, as imbalances can increase the risk of heart disease. By understanding how hormones impact heart health and implementing strategies to balance them, women can transform their heart health and reduce their risk of cardiovascular issues.

One of the essential hormones that affect heart health in women is estrogen. Estrogen helps to protect the heart by improving cholesterol levels, reducing inflammation, and promoting healthy blood vessel function. However, as women age and enter menopause, estrogen levels naturally decline, increasing the risk of heart disease. By focusing on hormone regulation through lifestyle changes, such as maintaining a healthy weight, exercising regularly, and managing stress, women can support their heart health and reduce the impact of hormonal changes.

Another vital hormone for heart health is progesterone. Progesterone helps to counterbalance the effects of estrogen and promote a healthy cardiovascular system. When progesterone levels are low, women may experience symptoms such as irregular heartbeats, high blood pressure, and increased risk of heart disease. By working with a healthcare provider to monitor hormone levels and implement hormone replacement therapy if needed, women can support their heart health and reduce the risk of cardiovascular issues.

In addition to estrogen and progesterone, other hormones such as cortisol and thyroid play a role in heart health. Chronic stress can lead to elevated levels of cortisol, which can contribute to inflammation, high blood pressure, and an increased risk of heart disease. By practicing stress-reducing techniques such as meditation, yoga, or deep breathing exercises, women can help regulate cortisol levels and support their heart health. Similarly, ensuring that thyroid hormones are balanced through proper nutrition, adequate sleep, and regular exercise can also benefit heart health.

Overall, by understanding the connection between hormone regulation and heart health, women in midlife can make positive changes to support their cardiovascular well-being. By focusing on lifestyle factors that promote hormone balance, working with healthcare providers to monitor hormone levels, and implementing strategies to reduce stress and support overall health, women can transform their heart health and reduce their risk of heart disease. The belev method provides valuable insights and strategies to help women achieve hormone balance and improve heart health, empowering them to take control of their well-being and live a heart-healthy life.

Tips for Maintaining Hormone Balance and Heart Health Long-term

Maintaining hormone balance and heart health long-term is crucial for women in perimenopause to ensure overall well-being and vitality. By following these tips, you can optimize your hormone levels and reduce your risk of heart disease.

First and foremost, it is important to prioritize a healthy diet rich in fruits, vegetables, whole grains, lean proteins, and healthy fats.

Avoiding processed foods, sugar, and excessive caffeine can help regulate hormone levels and support heart health. Incorporating foods high in omega-3 fatty acids, such as salmon, walnuts, and flaxseeds, can also help reduce inflammation and support cardiovascular health.

Regular exercise is another crucial component of maintaining hormone balance and heart health. Aim for at least 150 minutes of moderate-intensity aerobic activity per week and strength training exercises at least twice weekly. Exercise helps balance hormones, improves heart function, lowers blood pressure, and reduces risk factors for heart disease.

Managing stress is essential for hormone balance and heart health. Chronic stress can disrupt hormone levels and increase the risk of heart disease. Incorporating stress-reducing activities such as meditation, yoga, deep breathing exercises, and time in nature can help balance hormones and support cardiovascular health.

Finally, getting an adequate amount of quality sleep is crucial for hormone balance and heart health. Aim for 7-9 hours of uninterrupted sleep each night to allow your body to repair and restore hormone levels. Poor sleep can disrupt hormone balance, increase inflammation, and raise the risk of heart disease. Prioritizing these long-term tips for maintaining hormone balance and heart health can help perimenopausal women optimize their health and well-being. By making small, consistent changes to your diet, exercise, stress management, and sleep habits, you can support hormone balance and reduce your risk of heart disease. Consider a healthcare provider or hormone specialist for personalized recommendations tailored to your needs.

Resources for Women's Hormone Balance and Heart Health

In this section, you'll find suggested books and websites for delving deeper into women's hormone balance and cardiometabolic health. These resources can expand your knowledge on the subjects covered in this book and offer additional insights to aid you in achieving hormonal balance and enhancing heart health.

One highly recommended read is "The Hormone Cure" by Dr. Sara Gottfried. This book presents a thorough manual on comprehending and harmonizing hormones holistically. Dr. Gottfried offers practical tips on dietary adjustments, lifestyle modifications, and natural remedies to assist women in optimizing their hormonal well-being and enhancing their overall quality of life.

Another valuable resource is "The Wisdom of Menopause" by Dr. Christiane Northrup. This book delves into the physical and emotional transformations that occur during menopause, offering guidance on navigating this period with dignity and empowerment. Dr. Northrup's holistic approach to menopause underscores the significance of self-care, self-awareness, and self-compassion.

For those keen on delving into heart health and cardiometabolic well-being, we suggest exploring "Heart Solution for Women" by Dr. Mark Menolascino. This book presents scientifically backed strategies for preventing and reversing heart conditions in women, emphasizing personalized healthcare approaches, nutritional guidelines, and lifestyle adjustments. Dr. Menolascino's method for heart wellness addresses underlying hormonal imbalances and metabolic issues.

Besides books, various websites offer valuable information about women's hormone balance and cardiometabolic health. One such site is Hormone Health Network, which provides a range of resources on hormonal well-being, including articles, videos, and interactive tools to help women better understand their hormones and their impact on overall health. Another useful website is WomenHeart: The National Coalition for Women with Heart Disease, which offers support, education, and advocacy for women dealing with heart disease.

By delving into these suggested books and websites, you can better understand women's hormone balance and cardiometabolic health. This knowledge will empower you with the necessary tools to optimize your well-being. Remember that expertise holds power; the more you learn about your body and how to maintain its natural balance, the better prepared you'll be to lead a vibrant and healthy life.

Seeking Healthcare Professionals Specializing in Women's Hormone Balance and Cardiometabolic Health

As women grow older, hormone imbalances can significantly affect their overall health. Symptoms like hot flashes, mood swings, weight gain, and fatigue can be challenging to deal with. Thankfully, there are healthcare providers who specialize in women's hormone balance and cardiometabolic health ready to address these issues.

Thorough research is essential when looking for a healthcare professional specializing in women's hormone balance and cardiometabolic health. Seek out providers who have experience working with women in your age range and possess a solid understanding of the hormonal changes that occur during this phase of life. Ask for recommendations from friends, family, or trusted healthcare experts to steer you in the right direction.

Once you've identified a potential healthcare provider, arrange a consultation to discuss your concerns and objectives. Be ready to share a detailed medical history, including any symptoms you're currently dealing with and treatments you've previously undergone. This information will assist the provider in creating a customized treatment plan tailored to your needs and goals.

During your consultation, don't hesitate to ask about the provider's approach to women's hormone balance and cardiometabolic health. Please inquire about the types of treatments available, their success rates, and any potential side effects or risks involved. Feeling at ease and confident in your provider's skills and knowledge is crucial before proceeding with any treatment regimen.

In summary, discovering a healthcare professional specializing in women's hormone balance and cardiometabolic health can play a vital role in enhancing overall health and well-being.

Engage in thorough research, inquire actively, and collaborate with a professional who comprehends your individual requirements to empower yourself in managing your hormonal well-being and striving for ideal equilibrium and cardiovascular wellness. Do not hesitate to reach out for assistance and guidance—prioritizing your well-being and joy is of the utmost importance.

My gift to you - enclosed you will find my 12 week Belev Method guide, may you find it useful and as a resource to get you started and motivated. Stay consistent and persistent on your road to health and wellness.

Meet Dr. Isabel Bogdan, the owner and founder of Belev. co. With over 20 years as a women's health nurse practitioner and a doctorate in nursing practice, Dr. Bogdan's inspiration comes from a vision to intertwine traditional medicine with a holistic approach to transformational change. Isabel holds a 500 RYT yoga certification. Her comprehensive background includes certifications in functional medicine, yoga, caring for teens, young adults, and women of childbearing age, perimenopause, and menopause. Her specialty includes weight management, perinatal mental health, and aesthetics.

Dr. Bogdan is committed to empowering women with personalized integrative wellness plans, encompassing weight management, longevity medicine, and skin care. Her services are not bound by location, as they are available both virtually and in person. This adaptability has proven to be a boon, particularly in these challenging times. Her program is meticulously designed to address mindset, nutritional needs, metabolic function, essential movement, and aesthetics, all tailored to help women achieve their unique level of holistic wellness.

This same philosophy builds onto her design of belev.co, a women's health brand where the daily conversation involves sisterhood, community, mindset, and monthly women's health topics relevant to our needs throughout the lifespan. Dr. Bogdan said, "As time passes, women have entered my practice with more comorbidities than I've ever seen. I felt it was time to stop being a bystander and build a business where I could reach many via social media and Zoom. Where we gather to explore mindset, discuss nutritional needs, habit stack and bio hack to reach our ultimate goal of holistic wellness."

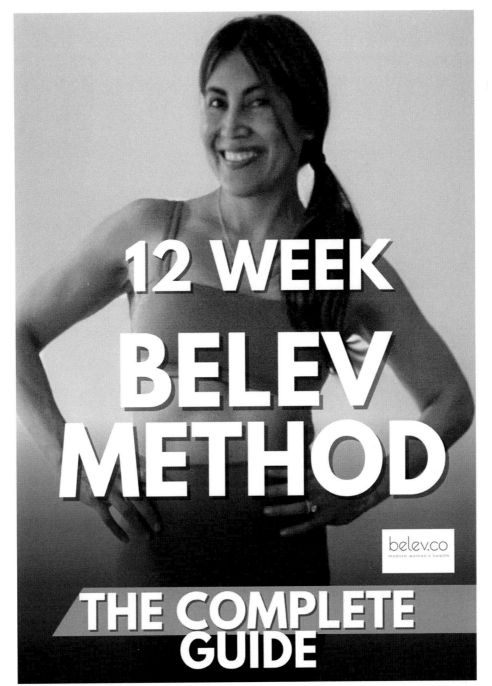

Disclaimer

Before beginning any exercise or nutrition program, it is important to consult with your healthcare provider.

The information provided by the personal trainer is for educational purposes only and is not intended to be a substitute for professional medical advice, diagnosis, or treatment.

This program does not replace working with a trainer or a licensed healthcare provider. The client assumes full responsibility for any risks, injuries, or damages, known or unknown, which may occur as a result of participating in the exercise or nutrition program.

The client acknowledges that exercise and nutrition programs involve a risk of injury, including but not limited to, heart attacks, muscle strains, sprains, broken bones, and other injuries. The client assumes all risks associated with participating in the exercise and nutrition program.

Belev, LLC is not responsible for any loss, injury, or damage sustained by the client while participating in the exercise or nutrition program. The client acknowledges that they have been advised to seek medical advice before beginning any exercise or nutrition program and to inform the personal trainer of any changes in their medical condition.

By participating in the exercise and nutrition program, the client acknowledges that they have read, understood, and agree to the terms of this disclaimer.

Contents

Welcome

Welcome to the 12 Week Belev Method: The Complete Guide!

This program is designed to help you achieve your fitness goals and transform your body in just 12 weeks. With a combination of strength training, high-intensity interval training (HIIT), and nutrition guidance, this program is guaranteed to challenge you and push you to your limits.

Whether you are a beginner or an experienced fitness enthusiast, the 12 Week Belev Method is tailored to meet your individual needs and help you reach your full potential.

So get ready to sweat, work hard, and see results like never before!

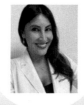

Isabel Bogdan

DNP, WHNP
I am specialized in women's health and hopeful this programming will help meet your weight management goals

✉ isabelbogdan@belev.co   🐦 isabel_bogdan
🌐 www.belev.co   📷 @drisabelbogdan

The complete overview

Let's take a further look into what 'fat' actually is, what it's used for and ultimately how to get rid of it. Fat plays many important roles inside the body including energy storage, regulating blood sugar levels, storage of certain vitamins and immune system function. But what does that even mean? Well, it means our body can run optimally when we have some fat on it.

Although it is important to have some fat, unfortunately, you can also have too much fat which can be bad for your health. There are a few ways to identify whether you're at risk of health problems that are linked to being overweight or having obesity such as girth measurements, skin calliper testing or body scan.

You can find a body fat percentile graph on the internet which shows the position and category of your body based on a few variables such as body type, heredity, age, activity and gender.

In this program, you are going to learn how you can effectively work smarter and not harder when it comes to staying in shape all year round.

LET'S START YOUR TRANSFORMATION

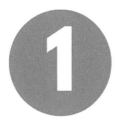

Nutrition

Food is more than just what we put in our mouths, it's actually information that tells our body what to do or what not to do.

When it comes to fat loss, nutrition plays a crucial role in achieving your goals. The key to successful fat loss is creating a caloric deficit, which means consuming fewer calories than your body burns each day. However, it's important to maintain a balanced and nutritious diet to ensure that your body is getting the necessary nutrients to function properly.

To support fat loss, it's recommended to consume a diet that is high in protein, as protein helps to keep you feeling full and can help preserve muscle mass while losing fat.

Meal planning and tracking your food intake can be helpful tools for ensuring that you are sticking to a calorie deficit and consuming a balanced diet. Additionally, drinking plenty of water, staying active, and getting enough sleep are all important factors in supporting fat loss.

We will touch more on these in the coming pages, but the most important thing to remember is that sustainable fat loss is a gradual process and should be approached with a long-term mindset. Fad diets and extreme restrictions are not sustainable or healthy, and can often lead to weight gain in the long run. A balanced, nutritious diet and a consistent exercise routine are key to achieving and maintaining healthy fat loss.

Energy Balance And Fat Loss

The foremost aspect of fat loss is establishing a calorie deficit. Without a calorie deficit, the body cannot lose fat. Unfortunately, a significant percentage of individuals are unaware of this fact and believe that consuming "healthy" foods is sufficient for weight loss.

It is important to note that a diet high in nutrient-dense foods is recommended, but it does not guarantee weight loss. All foods contain calories, which are our body's energy source. Similar to how fuel propels a car, food provides energy for our bodies to move.

To lose body fat, we must burn more calories than we consume, resulting in a negative energy balance, or a calorie deficit.

This creates a need for stored energy (body fat) to be used as fuel. The importance of other factors related to fat loss is relative to the foundation of the pyramid, which is a calorie deficit. Supplements, for example, have the least significance, while a calorie deficit is the most critical aspect.

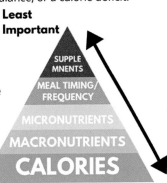

Least Important

SUPPLEMNENTS

MEAL TIMING/ FREQUENCY

MICRONUTRIENTS

MACRONUTRIENTS

CALORIES

Most Important

In conclusion, a calorie deficit is necessary to lose body fat.

Calculating Your Calorie Needs

We all need different amounts of food (energy) to be able to lose fat, build muscle or maintain weight. Below we're going to work out exactly how much you need.

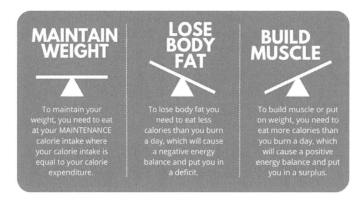

MAINTAIN WEIGHT

To maintain your weight, you need to eat at your MAINTENANCE calorie intake where your calorie intake is equal to your calorie expenditure.

LOSE BODY FAT

To lose body fat you need to eat less calories than you burn a day, which will cause a negative energy balance and put you in a deficit.

BUILD MUSCLE

To build muscle or put on weight, you need to eat more calories than you burn a day, which will cause a positive energy balance and put you in a surplus.

Step 1: Find Your BMR (Basal Metabolic Rate)

This refers to the minimum amount of energy or calories that the body requires to function properly while at rest. In other words, it is the number of calories needed to maintain basic bodily functions such as breathing, circulation, and organ function. BMR accounts for approximately 60-70% of the total calories that the body burns in a day, and it varies based on age, gender, body size, and genetics.

$$(10 \times \underline{\quad} \text{ kg}) + (6.25 \times \underline{\quad} \text{ cm}) - (5 \times \underline{\quad} \text{age}) - 161 = \text{calories}$$

For example: A female who **weighs 60kg**, is **170cm in height** and is **25 years old** would have a BMR of **1376 calories.**

Step 2: Find Your TDEE (Total Daily Energy Expenditure)

This refers to the total number of calories that an individual burns in a day, including the calories burned during daily activities and exercise. TDEE takes into account an individual's Basal Metabolic Rate (BMR), as well as the calories burned through physical activity and the thermic effect of food (the energy required to digest and process food). *Keep in mind that this is an estimate and may not be completely accurate for everyone. It's important to monitor your weight and adjust your calorie intake as needed based on your goals and progress.*

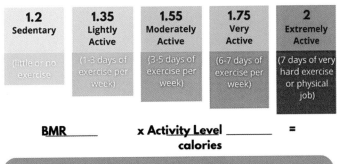

1.2 Sedentary	1.35 Lightly Active	1.55 Moderately Active	1.75 Very Active	2 Extremely Active
(little or no exercise)	(1-3 days of exercise per week)	(3-5 days of exercise per week)	(6-7 days of exercise per week)	(7 days of very hard exercise or physical job)

BMR _____ **x Activity Level** _____ **=** _____ calories

For example: A female who has a BMR of **1376 calories** and activity level of 1.55 would have a TDEE of **2132 calories.**

Step 3: Set Your Goal

Once you have calculated your TDEE, you can set your calorie goal by subtracting 300-500 calories from your TDEE. This will create a calorie deficit of 2100-7000 calories per week, which is equivalent to losing 0.6-1 pounds of fat per week. It's important to note that you should not aim to lose more than 1-2 pounds of fat per week, as this can be unsustainable and unhealthy.

For example: A female who has a TDEE of **2132 calories** and wants to aim to lose 500 grams of fat per week would need to set their calories at starting point of **1632 calories.**

Getting on top of your Macronutrients

Macronutrients, also known as "macros," are the three essential nutrients that provide energy and are required in large amounts in the human diet. The three macronutrients are:

Protein: Proteins are essential for building and repairing tissues in the body, including muscle, bone, and skin. They are found in foods such as meat, poultry, fish, beans, nuts, and dairy products. Proteins provide 4 calories per gram.

The amount of protein a person needs can vary depending on their age, sex, weight, physical activity level, and other factors. For example, athletes, bodybuilders, and people who are trying to lose weight or gain muscle may need more protein to support their goals. Recommended intake should be around 1.5-2g per kilogram of body weight

> Example: A female who weighs 60kg, is training consistently and is aiming for fat loss would be ideal to consume **120g of protein daily**, which is 480 calories.

Fat: Fats are also a source of energy for the body, but they are also important for many other functions, including hormone production, insulation of organs, and nutrient absorption. Fats are found in foods such as oils, nuts, seeds, butter, and fatty meats. Fats provide 9 calories per gram.

Similar to protein, the recommended daily intake of fat can vary depending on several factors, including age, sex, weight, and physical activity level. The Institute of Medicine suggests that adults should aim to get between 20% and 35% of their daily calorie intake from fat, with most of that coming from sources of healthy unsaturated fats, such as nuts, seeds, fatty fish, and oils like olive oil.

Example: For a female following a 1632 calorie diet, they should aim to consume **30% (54g) fat daily,** which is 490 calories.

Carbohydrates: Carbohydrates are the primary source of energy for the body. They are found in foods such as fruits, vegetables, grains, and dairy products. Carbohydrates provide 4 calories per gram.

The number of carbohydrates needed should make up 45-65% of your diet, otherwise can be made up with the remaining amount of calories after protein and fat has been considered.

Example: For a female following a 1632 calorie diet you do the sum: 1632 calories - (calories from protein 480 + calories from fat 490) = **662 calories (165g) allocated for carbs daily.**

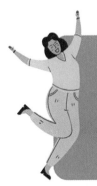

Daily Target Example:

1632 Calories
120g Protein
54g Fat
165g Carbohydrates

Food Choices For Each Macro

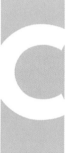

P		
Eggs	6g per Large egg
Milk	8g per 1 cup serving
Cottage cheese	14g per 1/2 serving
Steak	23g per 85g serving
Chicken breast	18g per 85g serving
Turkey breast	24g per 85g serving
Salmon	23g per 85g serving
Canned Tuna	22g per 85g serving
Peanut butter	8g per 2 tbsp
Whey Protein powder	24g per scoop

C		
Sweet Potatoes	20g per 100g
White Potatoes	13g per 100g
Brown Rice (Cooked)	23g per 100g
White Rice (Cooked)	25g per 100g
Oats	55g per 100g
Wholemeal Grain Bread	38g per 2 Slices
Whole Grain Pasta	41g per 1 Cup
Banana	27g per 1 Medium

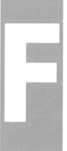

F		
Butter	12g per 1 tbsp
Avocado	15g per 100g
Extra Virgin Olive Oil	14g per 100g
Salmon	13g per 100g
Eggs	9g per 2 Large
Cheese	18g per 50g
Dark Chocolate	11g per 20g
Almonds	14g per 25g
Full-Fat Greek Yogurt	10g per 100g

Designing Your Own Meal Plan

Writing your own meal plan can be a helpful way to ensure that you are consuming a balanced and nutritious diet that aligns with your specific goals and preferences. Here are some general steps to consider when creating your own meal plan:

Determine your calories and macros: You should have already done this with the above steps.

Plan your meals: Begin by mapping out your meals for each day of the week. Start with breakfast, then move on to lunch, dinner, and snacks. Consider the foods you enjoy eating, as well as the macronutrient ratios you've chosen.

Example: Jane needs 1632 calories per day in order to start losing body fat, her work schedule is really busy so she decides to aim for breakfast, lunch, and dinner with 2 small snacks in between.

400 cal   **216 cal**   **400 cal**   **216 cal**   **400 cal**

Make a grocery list: Once you've determined your meals for the week, create a grocery list of the ingredients you'll need to prepare them. This can help you save time and money at the grocery store and ensure that you have everything you need for the week.

Track your progress: Keep track of your meals and progress by recording what you eat and how you feel each day. This can help you stay accountable and adjust your plan as needed.

Meal Frequency

The idea that eating smaller, more frequent meals can help with fat loss has been a popular one, but there is limited scientific evidence to support this notion. Some studies have suggested that increasing meal frequency may slightly increase metabolism, but the effect is small and may not translate to significant fat loss.

In general, the key to fat loss is creating a calorie deficit, which can be achieved through a variety of methods including reducing overall calorie intake, increasing physical activity, and managing stress levels. It's important to focus on consuming nutrient-dense foods that support overall health, rather than relying on meal frequency alone to achieve fat loss.

Ultimately, the best approach to meal frequency will depend on individual factors such as lifestyle, dietary preferences, and goals.

BREAKFAST RECIPES

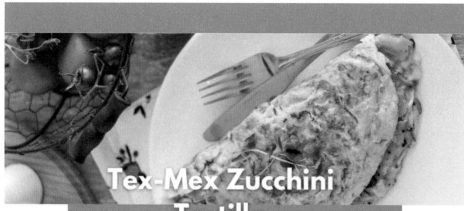

Tex-Mex Zucchini Tortilla

Serves: 2
Prep: 10 mins
Cook: 25 mins

Nutrition per serving:
377 kcal   22g Carbs
22g Fats   21g Protein

Ingredients

- 1 tbsp. olive oil
- 1 small potato, peeled, chopped
- 1 small onion, chopped
- ½ small zucchini, thinly sliced
- 6 eggs

Method

1. Heat oil in a non-stick pan and sear the potato and onion over medium-high heat, for about 4 minutes. Next, add the zucchini and sauté for another 4 minutes.

2. In a bowl, whisk eggs and season with salt and pepper. Transfer the vegetables from the pan into the bowl and mix well.

3. Using the same pan, add the egg mixture on low heat and make sure everything is evenly distributed. After about 3 minutes, run a spatula through the outer edges of the tortilla to make sure it does not stick to the pan.

4. After 8-10 minutes, flip the tortilla (this might take more or less, depending on heat, size and pan), using a plate over the pan. Slide the uncooked part back into the pan.

5. After another 5-6 minutes, the tortilla should be cooked, remove from heat and serve.

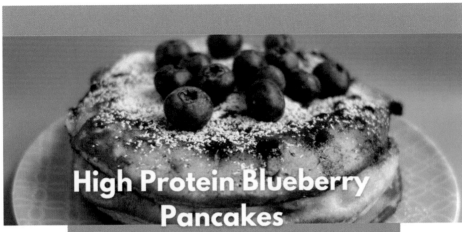

High Protein Blueberry Pancakes

 Serves: 1
Prep: 5 mins
Cook: 10 mins

 Nutrition per serving:
257 kcal   18g Carbs
5g Fats   36g Protein

Ingredients

- 1/4 cup liquid egg whites (around 4 eggs)
- 1 scoop (25g) of vanilla whey powder
- 1/2 banana, mashed
- almond milk, if needed
- 1/4 cup (25g) fresh or frozen blueberries
- ½ tsp. coconut oil

Method

1. Whisk together the egg whites and protein powder.

2. Stir in the mashed banana and add the blueberries. If the pancake mixture seems too thick, add a splash of almond milk to thin it.

3. Heat the coconut oil in a pan to low-medium. Pour in the pancake mixture and cook until little bubbles form (about 5 minutes).

4. Make sure the pancake has set enough before you try flipping it, then flip over. Cook the pancake for another 2-3 minutes.

5. You can also make 3 small pancakes instead of 1 large.

6. Serve with your favourite toppings.

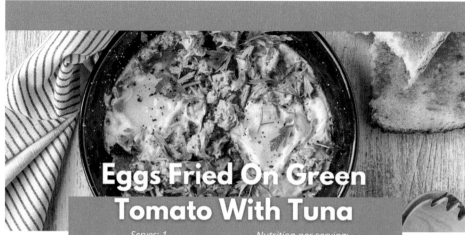

Eggs Fried On Green Tomato With Tuna

Serves: 1
Prep: 5 mins
Cook: 5 mins

Nutrition per serving:
307 kcal   8g Carbs
15g Fats   32g Protein

Ingredients

- 1 large green tomato
- 1 tsp. coconut oil
- 2 eggs
- 3 oz. (80g) tuna in brine
- a pinch of oregano
- a pinch of chili flakes
- parsley, chopped, to serve

Method

1. Peel the tomato and chop into cubes.

2. Heat the oil in a small frying pan, add the chopped tomato and fry over a high heat for about 3 minutes.

3. Create 2 gaps in the tomato and break the eggs into them. Season with salt and pepper.

4. Arrange pieces of Tuna on top. Then sprinkle with dried oregano and optionally chili flakes.

5. Fry for a further 3 minutes or until the egg whites are cooked. Serve with fresh parsley

Tips:
- Replace tuna with feta or Gorgonzola cheese
- For an extra carbohydrate boost serve with toasted bread or millet as a gluten-free option

LUNCH/ DINNER

RECIPES

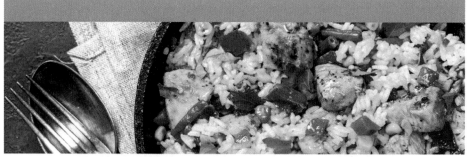

Louisiana Chicken With Veg Rice

 Serves: 3
Prep: 10 mins
Cook: 25 mins

 Nutrition per serving:
503 kcal   55g Carbs
13g Fats   40g Protein

Ingredients

- 1 tbsp. coconut oil
- 3 large carrots, sliced
- 2 peppers, sliced
- 4 spring onions, sliced
- 1 lb. (500g) chicken breast
- 2 tsp. Cajun seasoning
- 1 tbsp. tomato purée
- 1 lb. (500g) cooked rice

Method

1. Heat the oil in a large pan over medium heat. Add the carrots, peppers and white parts of the spring onions. Sauté for 10 minutes until the vegetables start to soften.

2. Add in the chicken breast, season with salt and pepper and cook for 10 minutes, until browned

3. Add the Cajun seasoning and tomato purée then stir well. Add in the cooked rice along with 4 tbsp. of water.

4. Stir well to combine all of the ingredients and heat for about 3-4 minutes.

5. Sprinkle with the green parts of the spring onion and serve.

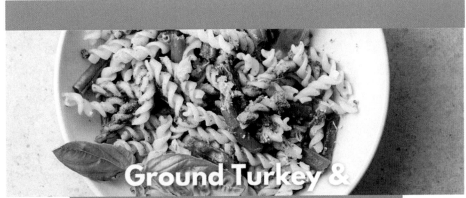

Ground Turkey & Green Bean Pasta

Serves: 2
Prep: 10 mins
Cook: 15 mins

Nutrition per serving:
491 kcal   53g Carbs
12g Fats   44g Protein

Ingredients

• 4 oz. (120g) whole-wheat pasta
• 1lb. ground turkey
• 4 spring onions
• 2 cloves garlic
• 1 tbsp. coconut oil
• 2 tbsp. soy sauce
• 1/3 cup (80ml) chicken stock
• 100g green beans, fresh

Method

1. Cook the pasta according to instructions on the packaging. Cut the beef into thin slices.

2. Slice the spring onions diagonally into 1-1.5 inch pieces. Peel and slice the garlic.

3. Heat the oil in a large pan over medium-high heat and cook on the turkey for about 3 minutes, then transfer onto a plate and drizzle with soy sauce.

4. Add the garlic and spring onion to the same pan and cook for about 3 minutes, until spring onions start to soften.

5. Return the turkey and soy sauce into the pan and add the hot stock and green beans. Cook for another 2-3 minutes, then add the cooked pasta, stir now and then for about 2 minutes.

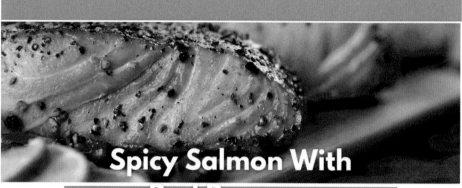

Spicy Salmon With Red Peppers

Serves: 2
Prep: 10 mins
Cook: 15 mins

Nutrition per serving:
491 kcal   53g Carbs
12g Fats   44g Protein

Ingredients

- 12 oz. (340g) salmon steak
- 4 tsp. plus 3 tbsp. soy sauce
- 1 tbsp. rice wine
- 3 tsp. buckwheat flour
- 2 tsp. coconut oil
- 1 large onion, sliced into strips
- 1 red bell pepper, sliced into strips
- 1/2 tsp. black pepper
- crushed red pepper flakes, to taste

Method

1. Place the salmon onto oiled pan lightly salted with pepper. Place in a bowl and add 4 tsp of soy sauce, 1 tbsp. of rice wine, 1 tsp. buckwheat flour and season with freshly ground black pepper.

2. In a small bowl, mix 3 tbsp. soy sauce, 1 tbsp. water and 2 tsp. buckwheat flour, then set aside. Then heat 1 tsp oil in a pan on high heat.

4. Add the salmon and cook for around 5 minutes on each side letting the salmon brown. Serve salmon on side dish.

5. Add the remaining 1 tsp. of oil to the pan, add the peppers and onions and cook about 4-5 minutes. Add the earlier prepared sauce and red pepper flakes (optional). Stir fry about 30-60 seconds on medium heat until slightly thickened.

6. Serves with rice or quinoa (not included in nutrition info per serving).

SNACK IDEAS

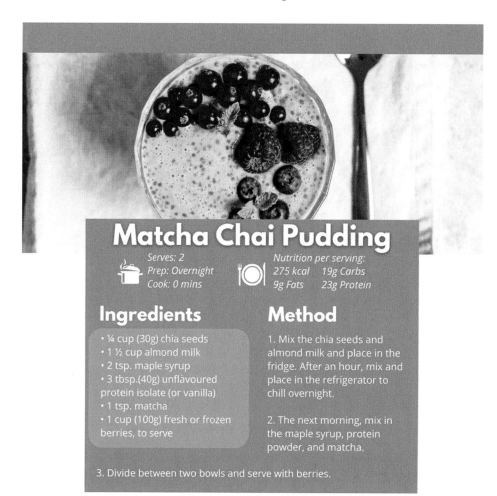

Matcha Chai Pudding

Serves: 2
Prep: Overnight
Cook: 0 mins

Nutrition per serving:
275 kcal   19g Carbs
9g Fats   23g Protein

Ingredients

- ¼ cup (30g) chia seeds
- 1 ½ cup almond milk
- 2 tsp. maple syrup
- 3 tbsp.(40g) unflavoured protein isolate (or vanilla)
- 1 tsp. matcha
- 1 cup (100g) fresh or frozen berries, to serve

Method

1. Mix the chia seeds and almond milk and place in the fridge. After an hour, mix and place in the refrigerator to chill overnight.

2. The next morning, mix in the maple syrup, protein powder, and matcha.

3. Divide between two bowls and serve with berries.

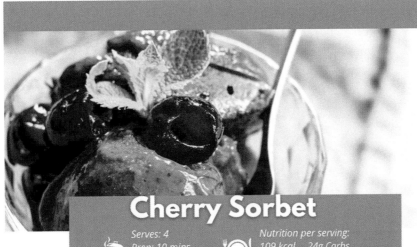

Cherry Sorbet

Serves: 4

Prep: 10 mins
Cook: 60 mins

Nutrition per serving:
109 kcal   24g Carbs
1g Fats   2g Protein

Ingredients

- 1 ¾ cups (400g) frozen pitted cherries
- 2 tbsp. honey
- 1 tbsp. lemon juice
- 4 tbsp. vanilla or plain greek yogurt
- 4 tbsp. water
- mint leaves, to serve

Method

1. Blitz the frozen cherries in a food processor or high speed blender with the honey, 1 tbsp. lemon juice, 4 tbsp. yogurt and 4 tbsp. water until smooth.

2. Spoon into a freezer-proof container then freeze for 1hr.

3. Scoop out the sorbet into serving glasses, top with mint and serve imminently.

4. The ingredients will make approx. 8 scoops of sorbet (2 per serving).

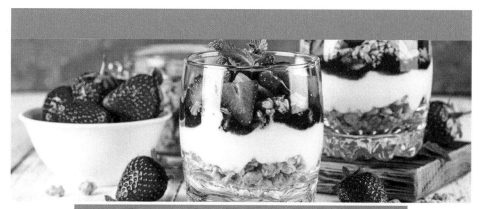

Protein Fruit Bowl

Serves: 2
 Prep: 10 mins
Cook: 0 mins

 Nutrition per serving:
250 kcal   30g Carbs
4g Fats   25g Protein

Ingredients

For the Mango Bowl:
• 7 oz. (200g) plain yogurt
• ¼ mango, chopped
• 1 tbsp. granola

For the Strawberry Bowl:
• 7 oz. (200g) plain yogurt
• 5 strawberries, halved
• ½ banana, sliced
• 1 tbsp. coconut chips

Method

1. Spoon the plain yogurt into serving bowls or glasses. Garnish with the toppings and serve.

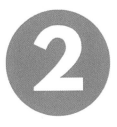

Exercise

The most important factor for fat loss is creating a calorie deficit. This can be achieved by burning calories through exercise, while also maintaining a healthy diet.

Here are few different types of training we can consider:

Cardiovascular exercise: Cardio is a great way to burn calories and increase your heart rate. Examples include running, cycling, swimming, and dancing.

High-intensity interval training (HIIT): HIIT workouts are a great way to burn a lot of calories in a short amount of time. These workouts involve short bursts of high-intensity exercise followed by brief rest periods. HIIT workouts can also help increase your metabolism and burn fat for hours after the workout is over.

Strength training: Strength training can help increase muscle mass, which can in turn help increase your metabolism and burn more calories. Aiming for strength-training sessions, focusing on compound exercises that target multiple muscle groups, such as squats, deadlifts, and bench presses - can ensure you're not only dropping body fat, but maintain muscle tissue.

Circuit training: Circuit training involves performing a series of exercises with little to no rest in between. This can help keep your heart rate elevated while also building strength and endurance.

CARDIO PYRAMID

Cardio can be a useful tool to incorporate into a weight training program for fat loss. One way to use cardio effectively is to perform it after weight training. This can help to maximise fat-burning potential, as weight training depletes glycogen stores, making your body more likely to turn to fat as a fuel source during cardio. The key is to find the balance of exercise that works for you!

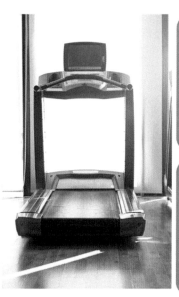

Beginners Incline Work

Begin speed 3, incline 4 - 5 minutes
speed 3, incline 8 - 5 minutes
speed 3, incline 12 - 10 minutes
speed 3, incline 8 - 5 minutes
speed 3, incline 4 - 5 minutes

Gradually increasing speeds and incline

Walk / Sprint / Jog

1. Begin speed 4, incline 8 - 5 minutes
2. speed 6, incline 2 - 5 minutes
3. speed 8, incline 0 - 1 minutes
4. speed 4, incline 8 - 1 minutes
5. speed 6, incline 2 - 2 minutes
Repeat steps 3, 4, 5 x 5 total 20 minutes
Bring speed to 4, incline 8 - 5 minutes

What We're Going To Focus On

Strength Training & Equipment

As I mentioned, there are various types of exercise that can assist with fat loss and keeping in shape. In my eyes there is definitely a hierarchy order as to what should be focused on more and what should be focused on less to see the best results.

In this program, we're going to focus on the most efficient form of exercise to burn fat and maintain muscle which is strength training.

Strength training will help maintain muscle mass, which can in turn increase your metabolism and help you burn more calories at rest. Additionally, strength training can help improve insulin sensitivity and help preserve muscle mass while you're losing weight, which can help prevent a drop in metabolism as you lose weight.

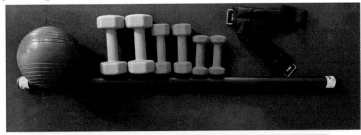

STYLE - PYRAMID

USE THE MODIFIED PYRAMID SYSTEM; include 15 second rests MAX in between sets - adding 2 lbs additional weight as you feel stronger to mitigate plateu effect

SET 1 - 12 repetitions, 3 lbs
SET 2 - 10 repetitions, 5 lbs
SET 3 - 6 to 8 repetitions, 8 lbs

Warming Up & Stretching

Warming up and stretching before weight training is important to help prevent injury and improve performance. A proper warm-up should gradually increase your heart rate, increase blood flow to the muscles, and prepare the body for the workout ahead. This can include light cardio, such as jogging or cycling, or dynamic stretching, such as leg swings or arm circles.

It's important to listen to your body and adjust your warm-up and stretching routine as needed. If you have any specific injuries or concerns, it's a good idea to consult with a specialist or healthcare provider for guidance on the best warm-up and stretching routine for your individual needs.

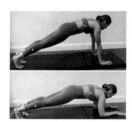

Runners Lunge Twist

Bodyweight Push Ups

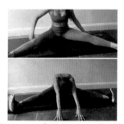

Runners Lunge Stretch

Forward Hammy & Glute Stretch

Weekly Workout Split

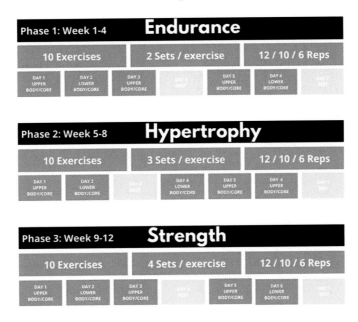

Phase 1: Week 1-4	Endurance		
10 Exercises	2 Sets / exercise		12 / 10 / 6 Reps

| DAY 1 UPPER BODY/CORE | DAY 2 LOWER BODY/CORE | DAY 3 UPPER BODY/CORE | DAY 4 REST | DAY 5 UPPER BODY/CORE | DAY 4 LOWER BODY/CORE | DAY 7 REST |

Phase 2: Week 5-8	Hypertrophy		
10 Exercises	3 Sets / exercise		12 / 10 / 6 Reps

| DAY 1 UPPER BODY/CORE | DAY 2 LOWER BODY/CORE | DAY 3 REST | DAY 4 LOWER BODY/CORE | DAY 5 UPPER BODY/CORE | DAY 6 UPPER BODY/CORE | DAY 7 REST |

Phase 3: Week 9-12	Strength		
10 Exercises	4 Sets / exercise		12 / 10 / 6 Reps

| DAY 1 UPPER BODY/CORE | DAY 2 LOWER BODY/CORE | DAY 3 UPPER BODY/CORE | DAY 4 REST | DAY 5 UPPER BODY/CORE | DAY 6 LOWER BODY/CORE | DAY 7 REST |

DAY 1 | UPPER BODY

Bicep Curls

INSTRUCTIONS

1) Get into position. Stand tall, with your feet hip-width apart. Hold a dumbbell in each hand, with your arms fully extended down by your sides and palms facing forward.
2) Engage your core muscles and tighten your abs to keep your body stable during the exercise. Perform the curling motion. When you reach the top, make sure your forearms are vertical and the weights are close to your shoulders. Pause briefly at this point to engage those biceps.
3) Lower with control.
4) Repeat for reps; Do the desired number of repetitions with form. Remember to breathe while performing each rep.

SETS x REPS	3 X12	WEIGHTS	WK 1	WK 2	WK 3	WK 4

LAT PULLDOWN

INSTRUCTIONS

1) Begin by holding dumbbells in each hand
2) Next hold the weight with an open grip ensuring your hands are slightly wider, than shoulder width apart. Pull the weight down towards your chest while maintaining a back and activating your lats.
3) Then gently return to the position focusing on controlling the motion throughout.

SETS x REPS	3 x 12	WEIGHTS	WK 1	WK 2	WK 3	WK 4

SINGLE ARM DUMBBELL ROW & FLY

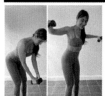

INSTRUCTIONS

1) Begin by standing, holding a dumbbell in each hand. Bend at your hips while keeping your back straight. Pull the dumbbells towards your body, squeezing your shoulder blades together. Lower them down.
2) Continue with dumbbell flies, holding a dumbbell in each hand and arms extended over your chest.
3) Lower the dumbbells out to the sides in an arc, feeling a stretch in your chest, then bring them up to the starting position while focusing on working the chest muscles throughout the exercise.

SETS x REPS	3 x 12	WEIGHTS	WK 1	WK 2	WK 3	WK 4

SINGLE DUMBBELL ROWS

INSTRUCTIONS

1) Lean forward at the waist with a dumbbell in each hand, then lift the weight towards your hip, bringing your shoulder blades closer together at the peak of the motion.
2) This exercise is great for developing strength and muscle mass in your back, which helps improve your posture and stability.

SETS x REPS	3 x 12	WEIGHTS	WK 1	WK 2	WK 3	WK 4

SKULLCRUSHERS (TRICEPS)

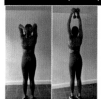

INSTRUCTIONS

1) Stand with your feet shoulder-width apart, holding a dumbbell with an overhand grip in each hand.
2) Bring the dumbbells up to shoulder height, elbows bent, and palms facing each other.
3) Engage your core for stability and ensure your back is straight.
Keeping your upper arms stationary, slowly extend your elbows to straighten your arms, lowering the dumbbells behind your head.
4) Pause briefly when your arms are parallel to the ground, then reverse the movement by bending your elbows to bring the dumbbells back to the starting position.

SETS x REPS	3 x 12	WEIGHTS	WK 1	WK 2	WK 3	WK 4

DAY 2 | LOWER BODY

PLIE SQUAT

INSTRUCTIONS

1) Position yourself with your feet set apart wider, than the width of your shoulders and heels touch toes outward. Hold a barbell on your upper back with a grip.
2) Maintain a strong back. Lift your chest as you lower your body by bending your knees and pushing your hips back until your thighs are at least parallel to the ground. Push up through your heels to come back, to the position making sure to engage your glutes at the peak of the movement.
3) Repeat this sequence for the desired number of reps focusing on maintaining form and alignment throughout the activity.

			WK 1	WK 2	WK 3	WK 4
SETS x REPS	3 x 12	**WEIGHTS**				

REVERSE DUMBBELL LUNGES

INSTRUCTIONS

1) Stand with dumbbells in both hands hanging down your sides.
2) Extend one leg back and lower your body on the other leg until knee of rear leg is almost in contact with floor.
3) Return to original standing position.
4) Make sure your torso is straight during the whole exercise.

			WK 1	WK 2	WK 3	WK 4
SETS x REPS	3 x 12	**WEIGHTS**				

BARBELL PULSE SQUATS

INSTRUCTIONS

Barbell pulse squats involve pulsing or bouncing at the bottom of a squat to engage the muscles more intensely. To perform them:
1. Start by holding a barbell across your upper back with an overhand grip and standing with feet shoulder-width apart.
2. Descend into a squat, then pulse up and down slightly while maintaining tension in your legs and core, before returning to the starting position.
3. Incorporate these controlled pulses to add an extra challenge and increase muscle activation during your squat routine.

			WK 1	WK 2	WK 3	WK 4
SETS x REPS	3 x 12	**WEIGHTS**				

LEG EXTENSION AND LIFT

INSTRUCTIONS

1) Begin by getting in table top with your knees at hip width and your hands at the front of the mat.
2) Raise one leg straight behind you, ensuring it stays parallel to the ground, and lift
3) Return to the starting position and switch sides for a rounded workout that tones and strengthens your legs.

			WK 1	WK 2	WK 3	WK 4
SETS x REPS	3 x 12	**WEIGHTS**				

BENT KNEE UPS

INSTRUCTIONS

1) Begin on all fours with your hands directly under your shoulders and your knees directly under your hips, maintaining a neutral spine.
2) Keeping your core engaged for stability, lift one knee off the ground while maintaining a 90-degree bend in the leg, bringing your heel towards the ceiling.
3) Squeeze your glutes at the top of the movement, then lower your knee back down to the starting position with control. Repeat for the desired number of repetitions on one side before switching to the other leg. This exercise effectively targets and strengthens the glute muscles while also engaging the core for stability and balance.

			WK 1	WK 2	WK 3	WK 4
SETS x REPS	3 x 12	**WEIGHTS**				

DAY 3 | CORE

BRIDGE SINGLES AND PULSE

INSTRUCTIONS

1) Begin by lying on your back with your knees bent and feet flat on the floor, hip-width apart.
2) Lift your hips off the ground by pressing through your heels and squeezing your glutes, forming a straight line from your shoulders to your knees.
3) Once in the bridge position, lift one leg off the ground and extend it straight out in front of you while maintaining the bridge position with your other leg. Then, pulse your hips up and down slightly while keeping the extended leg lifted, focusing on engaging your glutes. Return the extended leg to the floor and repeat the movement on the other side for a balanced workout. This exercise effectively targets and strengthens the glute muscles while also engaging the core and hamstrings.

SETS x REPS	3 x 12	WEIGHTS	WK 1	WK 2	WK 3	WK 4

CRUNCH CURL SIT UP

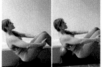

INSTRUCTIONS

1) Start by lying on your back with your knees bent and feet flat on the floor, hip-width apart.
2) Place your hands behind your head, elbows pointing out to the sides, and engage your core muscles.
3) Lift your head, neck, and shoulders off the ground by contracting your abdominal muscles, aiming to bring your chest towards your knees. Lower back down with control to complete one repetition. Repeat for the desired number of repetitions, focusing on maintaining proper form and breathing throughout the movement.

SETS x REPS	3 x 12	WEIGHTS	WK 1	WK 2	WK 3	WK 4

OBLIQUE TWIST AND CRUNCH

INSTRUCTIONS

1) Begin by lying on your back with your knees bent and feet flat on the floor, hip-width apart.
2) Place your hands behind your head, elbows pointing out to the sides, and engage your core muscles.
3) Lift your head, neck, and shoulders off the ground while simultaneously twisting your torso to one side, aiming to bring your opposite elbow towards your opposite knee. Lower back down with control and repeat the movement on the other side to complete one repetition. Alternate sides for the desired number of repetitions, focusing on engaging the oblique muscles and maintaining proper form throughout the exercise.

SETS x REPS	3 x 12	WEIGHTS	WK 1	WK 2	WK 3	WK 4

LOWER AB LIFTS

INSTRUCTIONS

1) Lie flat on your back with your legs extended and your arms by your sides.
2) Engage your core muscles and lift your legs off the ground, keeping them straight or slightly bent at the knees.
3) Slowly lower your legs towards the ground, stopping just before they touch, then raise them back up to the starting position. Repeat for the desired number of repetitions, focusing on using your lower abdominal muscles to control the movement and avoid arching your back.

SETS x REPS	3 x 12	WEIGHTS	WK 1	WK 2	WK 3	WK 4

UPPER CORE CRUNCH

INSTRUCTIONS

1) Lie flat on your back with your knees bent and feet flat on the floor, hip-width apart.
2) Place your hands behind your head, elbows pointing out to the sides, and engage your upper abdominal muscles.
3) Lift your head, neck, and shoulders off the ground by contracting your upper abdominal muscles, aiming to bring your chest towards your knees. Lower back down with control to complete one repetition. Repeat for the desired number of repetitions, focusing on maintaining proper form and avoiding pulling on your neck with your hands.

SETS x REPS	3 x 12	WEIGHTS	WK 1	WK 2	WK 3	WK 4

Tracking Sheet

DAY 1 REFLECTIONS	SLEEP	ENERGY	WATER	MOOD
	HRS	/10	/LITRES	/10

DAY 2 REFLECTIONS	SLEEP	ENERGY	WATER	MOOD
	HRS	/10	/LITRES	/10

DAY 3 REFLECTIONS	SLEEP	ENERGY	WATER	MOOD
	HRS	/10	/LITRES	/10

DAY 4 REFLECTIONS	SLEEP	ENERGY	WATER	MOOD
	HRS	/10	/LITRES	/10

DAY 5 REFLECTIONS	SLEEP	ENERGY	WATER	MOOD
	HRS	/10	/LITRES	/10

DAY 6 REFLECTIONS	SLEEP	ENERGY	WATER	MOOD
	HRS	/10	/LITRES	/10

DAY 7 REFLECTIONS	SLEEP	ENERGY	WATER	MOOD
	HRS	/10	/LITRES	/10

recommended supplements

The supplement industry is a massive business, and there seems to be a new product every second day which can be daunting for consumers to try to find the perfect one.

Buying supplements is a tricky process, so knowing exactly what the product will do and if it'll be necessary towards your goals will keep your bank account healthy and give you some piece of mind.

Here are some supplement recommendations

creatine

Creatine is a combination of 3 amino acids that is produced inside the body and also found in certain meats. Using creatine may boost your ATP energy levels which benefits activity levels involving short, fast, explosive movements.

multi-vitamin and omega 3's

Multivitamins are an array of different vitamins that you would usually find in food. Depending on your body, you may not be absorbing enough nutrients from your food which is why some people supplement with a good multivitamin.

protein powder

Protein powder is a dietary supplement that can be used to increase protein intake, which is important for muscle growth, repair, and overall health.

SLEEP & RECOVERY

Getting adequate sleep is important for overall health and can also support fat loss goals. Lack of sleep can disrupt hormones involved in appetite regulation, leading to increased hunger and cravings for unhealthy foods, and can also negatively impact metabolism and energy levels, making it harder to stick to healthy habits.

Research has shown that getting enough sleep (generally 7-9 hours per night) can support fat loss efforts by promoting healthy hormone levels and reducing cravings for unhealthy foods. In addition, getting adequate sleep can support recovery from exercise, which is an important component of fat loss.

Incorporating good sleep hygiene practices, such as establishing a consistent bedtime routine, avoiding caffeine and electronics before bed, and creating a comfortable sleep environment, can support quality sleep and overall health. It's important to prioritize adequate sleep along with other healthy lifestyle habits such as a healthy diet and regular physical activity for sustainable fat loss and optimal health.

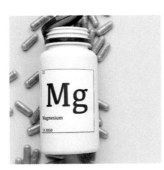

magnesium glycinate

Magnesium glycinate is known for its benefits for its "chill effects", better sleep and reducing anxiousness. It helps to relax the central nervous system and induce rest.

Thank You

Congratulations on completing the 12 Week Belev Method! I am thrilled to have been a part of your fitness journey and are so proud of all the hard work and dedication you put into achieving your goals. We hope that this program has helped you not only transform your body, but also your mindset and overall well-being.

As you move forward, I encourage you to keep up with the healthy habits you have developed during the program. Remember that fitness is a lifestyle, and the progress you have made in these 12 weeks is just the beginning. I invite you to continue your journey with me and explore other programs and resources we have to offer.

Thank you again for choosing the 12 Week Belev Method. We hope you enjoyed the program and are excited to see what you will accomplish in the future.
Keep up the great work!

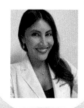

Isabel Bogdan, DNP, WHNP

Chat Further ...

Reach out anytime

Printed in the United States
by Baker & Taylor Publisher Services